SIMULATION IN NURSING EDUCATION

FROM CONCEPTUALIZATION TO EVALUATION

SECOND EDITION

Pamela R. Jeffries, PhD, RN, FAAN, ANEF

Editor

OUTCOMES

SIMULATION
DESIGN
CHARACTERISTICS

TEACHER
STUDENT
EDUCAT...
PRACTICES

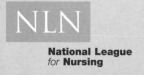

National League
for **Nursing**

National League for Nursing
61 Broadway
New York, NY 10006
212-363-5555 or 800-669-1656
www.nln.org

ISBN 978-1-934758-15-1

Cover design & art direction by Brian Vigorita

Figure 3-1 modified and included with permission of the National League for Nursing, New York

Figures 8-1, 8-2, and 8-3 courtesy of RCG Architects, Baltimore, MD

Figures 8-1, 8-2, and 8-3 included with permission of the University of Maryland School of Nursing, Baltimore, MD

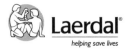

This publication has been proudly supported by Laerdal Medical Corporation.

The authors of this publication exercised full control over the content of each chapter.

Many specific products are mentioned throughout this publication. Such mention does not imply endorsement by the National League for Nursing.

Printed in the United States of America

DRC0812

SIMULATION IN NURSING EDUCATION

FROM CONCEPTUALIZATION TO EVALUATION
SECOND EDITION

TABLE OF CONTENTS

TABLE OF CONTENTS

List of Figures & Tables

LIST OF FIGURES & TABLES

Foreword to the Second Edition

In the six years since the first edition of this book was published, simulation, as a method to prepare health care professionals for a complex and changing health care environment, has become one of the most effective strategies used in both academic and service settings. Living up to its promise in the first edition, Simulation in Nursing Education has changed the way nurse educators teach and our students learn. The models for developing and using simulations proposed then have now been tested in all levels of nursing programs, and, as a result, there has been unprecedented growth in integration of simulations into all levels of the curriculum, development of well-resourced simulation laboratories and interdisciplinary simulation centers, and concomitant faculty development.

Widespread use of simulations has provided a mechanism to provide evidence on selected outcomes such as skill competency, clinical decision-making, teamwork, leadership, and confidence in the role of nurse. Correlation with similar benefits to clinical experience has resulted in local, and now national and international, studies to determine best practices for using simulations to complement, supplement, or replace certain low-frequency, high-risk learning experiences in clinical settings.

As nurse educators continue to address the ongoing changes in health care and nursing education and implement national reports to forge closer links between classroom learning and clinical practice, to work in teams, and to engage in interprofessional education and practice, simulation will be increasingly used to prepare nurses to provide safe care. Building on the foundations established in the first edition, and subsequent testing and development of simulation practices, this edition provides updated information that will be useful to both those who are experienced users of simulations and those now discovering the power of this strategy. This edition will continue to be the "go-to" resource for nurse educators and our colleagues.

Diane M. Billings, EdD, RN, FAAN
Chancellor's Professor Emeritus
Indiana University School of Nursing
Indianapolis, Indiana

PREFACE

It is hard to believe but it has been six years since the first edition of *Simulations in Nursing Education: From Conceptualization to Evaluation* was written. In the area of clinical simulations, much has changed since those early years when health professional educators were trying to figure out what to do with the manikin once it was out of the box. The results from the National League for Nursing and the Laerdal Corporation national, multi-site study that was conducted in 2003-2006 are still cited and impactful today. The multi-site study was completed to (a) develop and test models that nursing faculty can implement when using simulation in innovative ways to enhance student learning, (b) develop a cadre of nursing faculty who can use simulation in innovative ways to enhance student learning, (c) refine the body of knowledge about the use of simulation in nursing education, and (d) demonstrate the value of collaboration between the corporate and not-for-profit worlds.

From this former project, the first edition of this book was created and written by members of the project team and in some cases colleagues at project coordinator's schools. This second edition is again written by some of the same project team coordinators in addition to other simulation experts in the health care field today. Over the past six years many educators have focused their research on specific areas of simulation contributing to the body of knowledge and research in this area.

Today's health care reform and changing health needs create new competencies needed by our nursing graduates to care for all types of patients in diverse health care settings. Health care environments are complex, requiring health care professionals to have different skill sets than just a decade ago; health care professionals require high-tech, problem solving, and decision-making skills, as well as expert clinical knowledge, to care for the high-acuity patients in the acute care and other diverse settings. Nurse educators are responsible for preparing nursing graduates for the reality of health care practices to provide safe, competent, quality care.

The Future of Nursing: Leading Change, Advancing Health (2011) and other landmark reports have focused on nursing education and practice, highlighting the critical roles of nurse educators, practitioners, and the delivery of nursing care in complex health care environments. Key messages from the national reports require nurse educators to consider different teaching strategies and experiences to better prepare our graduates. Health care educators can use clinical simulations as one approach to create student-centered, experiential environments that engage and prepare the learner for real-world practice. The need to know more about how to design, develop, implement, and integrate simulations into nursing curricula is greater today than it was six years ago. Once exceptional, incorporating clinical simulations in a nursing curriculum is now commonplace.

The use of clinical simulations requires faculty from all types of programs and clinical institutions to learn the new pedagogy to obtain the optimal outcomes expected from using this educational methodology. This edition of *Simulations in Nursing Education: From*

Conceptualization to Evaluation has been developed to better prepare nurse educators for their role in developing, implementing, and evaluating the use of clinical simulations in the nursing curriculum and to supporting faculty to embracing this new pedagogy that is increasing in nursing education across different programs and across many nursing courses. When incorporating simulations into nursing education, nurse educators need to consider doing the following:

- Understanding the science of learning connected to the simulation pedagogy.

- Identifying the best practices that are emerging in the field of clinical simulations.

- Being prepared to deliver clinical simulations in an effective, efficient manner to optimize learning outcomes.

- Promoting a student-centered approach used in simulations versus teacher-centered seen in traditional clinical models.

- Facilitating clinical simulations that faculty are prepared for with the focus on their clinical expertise and practice.

- Providing a faculty development program for educators integrating simulations into the teaching-learning environment.

- Ensuring all faculty and students have an orientation to the simulation pedagogy, the simulators, the art of debriefing, and other expectations of clinical simulation when embarking on this experiential activity.

- Promoting the concept of collaborative partnerships and consortiums to work more efficiently, share resources, and to learn from each other.

- Developing an evaluation plan or process to measure learning outcomes and competencies required of the learner.

- Developing a plan of research to study the clinical simulation pedagogy to identify best practices and to contribute to the science of nursing education.

This second edition has been written to update the chapters from the first edition and to add new information in key areas that have risen to the forefront in clinical simulations. Two new chapters added to this edition include the expansion of the art of debriefing and a focus on integrating patient safety competencies into clinical simulations. Readers will learn more about advanced debriefing, different approaches, and what the evidence is showing us in the chapter entitled Debriefing an Essential Component for Learning in Simulation Pedagogy. In addition, with the national focus not only on health care reform but on promoting quality and safe patient care environments, another new chapter, entitled, Integrating the QSEN Competencies into Simulation, describes how the Quality in Safety for Education in Nursing (QSEN) competencies can be integrated into clinical simulation scenarios. Although this is a second edition, the book is still considered a foundational one, providing core, essential content to those educators who are just beginning their journey using clinical simulations whether they are in an academic setting or a clinical institution. The foundational content can get educators started by using this book as a guide and resource for developing, implementing, integrating, and evaluating clinical simulations in nursing education.

During this nursing education revolution, the use of clinical simulations is being considered a clinical redesign. Let's embrace this change and challenge; the time is right for new possibilities and opportunities in nursing education. The material in this book will help educators get started and take the next step in creating, implementing, integrating, and evaluating the use of this wonderful, experiential pedagogy that is creating a new model of clinical education.

Pamela R. Jeffries, PhD, RN, FAAN, ANEF

April 2012

Acknowledgments

We want to thank the contributors to the second edition of this book who graciously shared their expertise, wisdom, and passion for clinical simulations. In this second edition, we continue to value the work from the original chapter authors and thoughtfully respect the additions of our new contributors to the book. Also thanks to the reviewers who provided peer review of the book chapters. The reviews from colleagues are most helpful as we continue to strive to meet the needs of today's health care educators.

Thanks, too, to the National League for Nursing and the NLN publication team, Dr. Elaine Tagliareni, Janet Willhaus, and Anne Ganzer, for recognizing the need for a second edition. Many changes have occurred in the area of clinical simulations since the first printing in 2007. We especially thank Justine Fitzgerald for her editing and production expertise, organizational skills, and all the assistance she provided to the project. Thanks to Melissa Gillis, our copy editor, and to Laerdal Medical for having the vision to support development in nursing education focused on clinical simulations. Thanks to Brian Vigorita for cover design and layout. We would also like to thank Holly I. Powers, senior administrative coordinator, and Marie Brown, academic program manager, at Johns Hopkins University, for their organization and editing contributions.

We thank our families, colleagues, and nursing leaders for their continued support and encouragement throughout the project. In addition, thanks to all of the faculty, graduate, and doctoral nursing students who are embracing the notion of clinical simulations and studying the phenomena in your courses, thesis papers, and dissertations. Without the continued evidence in the area of simulations we cannot move forward. Your work and contributions are greatly appreciated.

P.R.J.

DEDICATION

This book is dedicated to all current and emerging nurse educators, who explore new ways to revolutionize nursing education through the use of clinical simulations. It is also dedicated to all nursing students as they immerse themselves in simulations or study simulation pedagogy through educational research. This book is also designed to stimulate current nurse educators and researchers to explore new, innovative teaching-learning strategies and to keep you engaged, interactive, and inspired to improve learning outcomes.

CHAPTER 1
USING SIMULATION IN NURSING EDUCATION

Mary L. Cato, MSN, RN

"I hear and I forget.

I see and I remember.

I do and I understand."

—Confucius

SIMULATION: PAST AND PRESENT

Simulation has become widely accepted as a valuable tool in nursing education. Due to a national nursing shortage, the growth of nursing education programs, and a shortage of clinical learning sites, many programs are utilizing simulation in various formats to help students learn the skills, roles, and responsibilities of the nurse. Advances in technology have facilitated the development of high-fidelity manikins that mimic human physiology and also audio/visual methods allowing simulations to be taped and transmitted to observers in real time and for later review. Educators in nursing and in other health care fields have been taking advantage of the technology and integrating simulation into pre-licensure, advanced practice, orientation, and continuing education programs.

Thanks to the increase in electronic resources, nurse educators have also been designing ways to share scenarios and simulation techniques with others across the country and around the globe. The National League for Nursing (NLN) Simulation Innovation Resource Center (SIRC) is an example of an online site providing that education and support (NLN, http://sirc.nln.org). There are also several professional organizations that offer resources via websites, listservs, and national and regional conferences. The International Nursing Association for Clinical Simulation and Learning (INACSL) publishes a monthly journal and is developing simulation standards for educators (www.inacsl.org). The Society for Simulation in Healthcare (SSiH) also publishes a journal and offers accreditation for simulation health care programs (https://ssih.org/). Workshops and courses are offered by many organizations across the country allowing faculty to gain knowledge and expertise in simulation.

As long-time educators may recall, the teaching of patient care skills has not always been dependent upon technology. Mrs. Chase was a low-fidelity, life-size adult manikin created by the M. J. Chase Company and first used at Hartford Hospital in 1911 for the practice of basic nursing skills (Herrmann, 1981). Task trainers that could be used to demonstrate and practice specific skills such as urethral catheter and gastric tube insertion, wound care, and injection administration were then developed. In the 1960s, the creation of Resusci Anne by the Laerdal Company provided users with a realistic airway which was used in the training of cardiopulmonary resuscitation. Computer controlled high-fidelity manikins with increasingly realistic physiology followed Resusci-Anne (Cooper & Taqueti, 2008). Educators now have access to a multitude of low-, medium-, and high-fidelity manikins, from a variety of manufacturers, that speak, breathe, and have heart and lung sounds, and also deliver babies, experience seizures, and produce various body fluids. As reported by Hovanscek (2007), "the introduction of affordable, portable, and versatile human patient simulators in the late 1990s transformed health care education and is the technology of the future for competency testing and continuing education" (p. 2).

It is not only the technology, however, that has spurred the increased use of simulation.

Nurse educators have long used strategies such as role-play to provide students with an opportunity to practice nursing, particularly for skills such as communication, health teaching, and assessment. Along with manikins, educators are using actors and standardized patients (SPs) in simulation. SPs are "people who may or may not be professional actors who are instructed on how to act as if they have a particular disease or condition in a given patient situation in a given health care setting" (Nehring & Lashley, 2010, p. 14). A very realistic or high-fidelity learning experience can be implemented through the use of SPs. Although some authors define simulation by the use of a manikin, a broader definition may be more useful when examining simulation's potential. When not limited by the technology, and defined as an "attempt to replicate some or nearly all of the essential aspects of a clinical situation so that the situation may be more readily understood and managed when it occurs for real in clinical practice" (Morton, 1995, p. 76), simulation has increased possibilities in health care education.

Describing Simulation

Typically, a simulation involves a student or group of students providing care for a patient who is represented by a manikin, an actor, or an SP, depending on the clinical situation. Often, simulation is an activity in which students participate in groups and are observed by faculty.

The patient care scenario is followed by a reflection, or debriefing period, during which the case is deconstructed and analyzed, and feedback is given to the participants by faculty and other students. Simulation is usually used to complement clinical learning that is done in patient care environments such as hospitals, clinics, long-term care centers, and community settings.

Creative instructors are designing simulations to meet the needs of learners in diverse settings. Simulations are being taped and watched from remote sites to engage more learners in the activity. Students are observing their own taped scenarios, reflecting on their actions, and evaluating their performances. Simulations are being implemented with multiple patients, requiring students to prioritize and manage their care in realistic ways. Nursing students are being given opportunities to care for simulated patients alongside multiple other disciplines, including physicians, respiratory therapists, and social workers, helping them adapt to the interprofessional nature of health care. These are only a few of the many ways in which simulation can be used in nursing education.

PREVALENCE OF SIMULATION IN NURSING EDUCATION

Nursing education literature substantiates the fact that simulation is becoming increasingly common as a clinical learning tool (Jeffries, 2007; Kaakinen & Arwood, 2009; Sinclair & Ferguson, 2009). In 2010, during phase 1 of a national, multi-site study of simulation in nursing education, the National Council of State Boards of Nursing (NCSBN) conducted a survey to assess the use of simulation in pre-licensure nursing programs in the United States. This large-scale study began with the mailing of 1,729 surveys to programs for registered nurse education, including associate, baccalaureate, and master's degree programs. The 62 percent response rate (1,060 surveys were completed) included data from every state in the country. Colleges, universities, and technical schools from both urban and rural areas were represented (Hayden, 2010).

Three types of simulation, as determined by fidelity, were defined for this survey, and they included not only the use of manikins, but SPs as well. Hayden (2010) defined high-fidelity simulation as a "patient-care scenario that uses a standardized patient or a full-body patient simulator that can be programmed to respond to affective and psychomotor changes, such as breathing chest action" (p. 52), and medium-fidelity simulation as a "patient-care scenario that uses a full-body simulator with installed human qualities such as breath sounds without chest rise" (p. 52). Hayden defined the third type of simulation as "task trainers," or "part of a manikin designed for a specific psychomotor skill, for example, an arm for IV insertion practice" (p. 52).

According to Hayden (2010), 87 percent of the respondents in the NCSBN study reported using high- or mid-fidelity simulation experiences in their programs, with 54 percent using simulation in five or more nursing courses. Simulation was used most frequently in courses teaching foundations of nursing and care of medical and surgical patients. Although assessment and psychomotor skills were listed as the focus of most simulations, faculty also reported using simulation for teaching behavioral skills such as communication, clinical decision-making, and interdisciplinary team training.

The NCSBN study results demonstrate that instructors across the country utilize and value simulation as a desired teaching strategy. Their approval is evident in the responses to a question about how much simulation should be used in nursing programs. Respondents were asked whether they believed their nursing education programs should be using more or less simulation. Eighty-one percent thought that using more simulation would be preferred, 18 percent believed they were using the right amount, and only three respondents believed they were using too much (Hayden, 2010).

Simulation is used more often for practice than for student evaluation in nursing. However, in current and future phases of the NCSBN study, the role and outcomes of simulation use will be explored, including an examination of simulation for high-stakes testing, such as licensure exams, certification, or performance appraisal (NCSBN, 2012). This may mean that, in the future, we will see an increase in the use of simulation for low-stakes assessment such as measuring progress toward course or programmatic goals and for high-stakes testing (Jeffries, Hovancsek, & Clochesy, 2005). The development of valid and reliable measurement tools and methods is critical, especially for high-stakes testing.

There is increasing evidence in the literature describing how simulation is used to promote learning in nursing and other health care professions. Simulation has been demonstrated as effective in improving student cognitive skills and critical thinking (Elfrink, Kirkpatrick, Nininger, & Schubert, 2010; Kaddoura, 2010), self-confidence and self-efficacy, (Blum, Borglund, & Parcells, 2010; Wagner, Bear, & Sander, 2009; Schoening, Sittner, & Todd, 2006; Sinclair & Ferguson, 2009), clinical judgment (Lasater, 2007), clinical skills and clinical performance (Alinier, Hunt, Gordon, & Harwood, 2006; Anderson & Warren, 2011; Meyer, Connors, Hou, & Gajewski, 2011), safe medication administration (Sears, Goldsworthy, & Goodman, 2010), and leadership skills (Reed, Lancaster, & Musser, 2009). As students graduate and enter the practice arena, simulation has been used to help them transition into professional practice (Chappy, Jambunathan, & Marnoch, 2010; Stefanski & Rossler, 2009). In the interest of patient safety, simulation is used to facilitate teamwork and communication both inter- and intra-professionally (Kuehster & Hall, 2010). Focusing on the affective domain, others have used simulation to promote learning in the areas of cultural diversity and caring (Eggenberger, Keller, & Locsin, 2010; Haas, Seckman, & Rea, 2010; Storr, 2010), nursing care at end-of-life (Hamilton, 2010; Smith-Stoner, 2009), and ethical decision-making (Gropelli, 2010).

Because it is a practice discipline, nursing must be taught not only in the classroom, but in clinical areas as well. Students need to practice the necessary skills, apply the knowledge learned, and incorporate the behaviors needed to practice nursing in a real environment. Simulation has been incorporated into nursing education because it allows students to "engage in the same critical thinking and clinical decision-making skills required in actual clinical practice" (Sinclair & Ferguson, 2009, p. 1). When utilized as a clinical learning activity, simulation builds upon what students know and allows them to demonstrate their knowledge and skills in a safe learning environment by providing "a wide range of experiences that are either too rare or too risky for novices to engage in using actual patients" (Hovancsek, 2007, p. 3). With support from faculty, simulation can help bridge the gap between the classroom and the patient care environment.

ADVANTAGES TO USING SIMULATION

As Hovancsek (2007) explained, "it is not enough for nurse educators to include simulation in their courses because it is popular, available, or 'trendy'" (p. 5). It is important to base simulation practices on learning theory and evidence of its effectiveness. Designing and implementing simulations to meet specific course and program objectives is vital in nursing education.

Using simulations, faculty can involve students in clinical situations they may not see or be allowed to participate in with actual patients, such as resuscitations or critical events like management of shock or anaphylaxis. An advantage in simulation is that "the instructor, preceptor, or staff nurse does not take over, as often happens on a clinical unit when students are mishandling a situation or having difficulty with a skill" (Hovancsek, 2007, p. 5). Ideally, simulations are planned at a level appropriate for students, and students have been given an opportunity to study and prepare for the simulation activity. Nevertheless, in simulation, students may make poor decisions, perform interventions ineffectively, or fail to respond to a patient situation. Instructors can use these situations as opportunities for student learning as they review the case and help students analyze what happened and why they responded in a certain way. Students can also gain increased expertise in professional communication as they receive and provide feedback in the debriefing that follows a simulation.

Challenges of Using Simulation

One of the greatest challenges of using simulation in nursing education is the expense. In some cases, the cost of a manikin is more than program budgets allow. All too often, funds that are obtained are used only for the manikin and there is no consideration of faculty training and time, environmental and space requirements, and support personnel. There is a risk of developing simulation programs based on equipment and technology without a plan for meaningful utilization and curricular integration (Seropian, Brown, Gavilanes, & Driggers, 2004).

It is critical that simulation users are prepared not only to operate the equipment, but also to understand the pedagogy that supports simulation. Research into the effectiveness and the transferability of knowledge to patient care will help nurse educators plan, implement, and integrate simulation activities into nursing curricula, and this research needs to be supported both programmatically and financially. Nursing care, and therefore nursing education, is complex and vital to patient outcomes in a multitude of situations. As Schiavenato (2009) explains, "the challenge in nursing education is not the integration of the human patient simulator in nursing curriculum but rather the reconceptualization of simulation as a teaching tool encompassing varied methods and a wealth of applications throughout the prenursing and nursing curricula" (p. 392).

SUMMARY AND CONCLUSION

As explained in the first edition of this book, simulation has unlimited potential as a teaching tool in nursing education. Although there has been a proliferation of simulation research over the past several years, continued research is necessary to help us understand how learning is achieved and how this learning can be transferred to patient care with "real" patients. The following chapters address multiple issues related to simulation. They will provide a theoretical framework for simulation and help educators design simulations and integrate them into curricula. They will explain how debriefing and guided reflection can be used to broaden and deepen the learning experience in simulation. And, they will examine the evaluation of simulation along with considerations for the use of simulation in the future of nursing education.

References

Alinier, G., Hunt, B., Gordon, R., & Harwood, C. (2006). Effectiveness of intermediate-fidelity simulation training technology in undergraduate nursing education. *Journal of Advanced Nursing, 54*(3), 359-369.

Anderson, J. M. & Warren, J. B. (2011). Using simulation to enhance the acquisition and retention of clinical skills in neonatology. *Seminars in Perinatology, 35*, 59-67. doi:10.1053/j.semperi.2011.01.004

Blum, C. A., Borglund, S., & Parcells, D. (2010). High-fidelity nursing simulation: Impact on student self-confidence and clinical competence. *International Journal of Nursing Education Scholarship, 7*(1), Article 18. doi:10:2202/1548-923X.2035

Chappy, S., Jambunathan, J., & Marnoch, S. (2010). Evidence-based curricular strategies to enhance BSN graduates' transition into practice. *Nurse Educator, 35*(1) 20-24.

Cooper, J. B. & Taqueti, V. R. (2008). A brief history of the development of manikin simulators for clinical education and training. *Postgraduate Medical Journal, 84*, 563-570. doi:10.1136/qshc.2004.009886

Eggenerger, T., Keller, K., & Locsin, R. C. (2010). Valuing caring behaviors within simulated emergent nursing situations. *International Journal for Human Caring, 14*(2), 23-29.

Elfrink, V. L., Kirkpatrick, B., Nininger, J., & Schubert, C. (2010). Using learning outcomes to inform teaching practices in human patient simulation. *Nursing Education Perspectives, 31*(2), 97-100.

Gropelli, T. M. (2010). Using active simulation to enhance learning of nursing ethics. *Journal of Continuing Education in Nursing, 41*(3), 104-105.

Haas, B., Seckman, C., & Rea, G. (2010). Incorporating cultural diversity and caring through simulation in a baccalaureate nursing program. *International Journal for Human Caring, 14*(2), 51-52.

Hamilton, C. A. (2010). The simulation imperative of end-of-life education. *Clinical Simulation in Nursing, 6*(4), e131-e138. doi:10.1016/j.ecns.2009.08.002

Hayden, J. (2010). Use of simulation in nursing education: National survey results. *Journal of Nursing Regulation, 1*(3) 52-57.

Hermann, E. K. (1981, October). Mrs. Chase: A noble and enduring figure. *American Journal of Nursing, 81*(10), 1836.

Hovancsek, M. T. (2007). Using simulation in nursing education. In P. Jeffries, (Ed.), *Simulation in nursing education: From conceptualization to evaluation.* New York, NY: National League for Nursing.

Jeffries, P.R. (2007). Simulations in Nursing Education: From Conceptulization to Evaluation. The National League for Nursing, New York: New York.

Jeffries, P. R., Hovancsek, M. T., & Clochesy, J. M. (2005). Using clinical simulations in distance education. In J. M. Novotny & R. H. Davis (Eds.), Distance education in nursing (2nd ed.) (pp. 83-99). New York, NY: Springer.

Kaakinen, J., & Arwood, E. (2009). Systematic review of nursing simulation literature for use of learning theory. *International Journal of Nursing Education Scholarship, 6*(1), Article 16. doi:10.2202/1548-923X1688

Kaddoura, M. A. (2010). New graduate nurses' perceptions of the effects of clinical simulation on their critical thinking, learning, and confidence. *Journal of Continuing Education in Nursing, 41*(11), 506-516.

Kuehster, C. R., & Hall, C. D. (2010). Learning from mistakes while building communication and teamwork. *Journal for Nurses in Staff Development, 26*(3), 123–127.

Lasater, K. (2007). High fidelity simulation and the development of clinical judgment: Students' experiences. *Journal of Nursing Education, 46*(6), 269-276.

Meyer, M. N., Connors, H., Hou, Q., & Gajewski, B. (2011). The effect of simulation on clinical performance. *Simulation in Healthcare, 6*(5), 269-277. doi:10.1097/SIH.0b013e318223a048

Morton, P. G. (1995). Creating a laboratory that simulates the critical care environment. *Critical Care Nurse, 16*(6), 76-81.

National Council of State Boards of Nursing. (2012). NCSBN National Simulation Study. In *https://www.ncsbn.org*. Retrieved July 5, 2012, from https://www.ncsbn.org/2094.htm.

National League for Nursing. (nd). Simulation Innovation Resource Center. In *http://sirc.nln.org/*. Retrieved July 5, 2012 from http://sirc.nln.org.

Nehring, W. M. & Lashley, F. R. (2010). *High-fidelity patient simulation in nursing education.* Sudbury, MA: Jones and Bartlett.

Reed, C. C., Lancaster, R. R., & Musser, D. B. (2009) Nursing leadership and management simulation creating complexity. *Clinical Simulation in Nursing,* 5(1), e17-e21.

Schiavenato, M. (2009). Reevaluating simulation in nursing education: Beyond the human patient simulator. *Journal of Nursing Education, 48*(7), 388-394. doi:10.3928/01484834-20090615-06

Schoening, A. M., Sittner, B. J., & Todd, M. J. (2006). Simulated clinical experience: Nursing students' perceptions and the educators' role. *Nurse Educator, 31*(6) 253-258.

Sears, K., Goldsworthy, S., & Goodman, W. M. (2010). The relationship between simulation in nursing education and medication safety. *Journal of Nursing Education, 49*(1), 52-55.

Seropian, M. A., Brown, K., Gavilanes, J. S., & Driggers, B. (2004). Simulation: Not just a manikin. *Journal of Nursing Education, 43*, 164-169.

Sinclair, B., & Ferguson, K. (2009). Integrating simulated teaching/learning strategies in undergraduate nursing education. *International Journal of Nursing Scholarship, 6*(1), 1-10. doi:10.2202/1548-923X1676

Smith-Stoner, M. (2009). Using high-fidelity simulation to educate nursing students about end-of-life care. *Nursing Education Perspectives, 30*(2), 115–120.

Stefanski, R. R., & Rossler, K. L. (2009). Preparing the novice critical care nurse: A community-wide collaboration using the benefits of simulation. *The Journal of Continuing Education in Nursing, 40*(10), 443-453.

Storr, G. B. (2010). Learning how to effectively connect with patients through low-tech simulation scenarios. *International Journal for Human Caring, 14*(2), 36-40.

Wagner, D., Bear, M., & Sander, J. (2009). Turning simulation into reality: Increasing student competence and confidence, *Journal of Nursing Education, 48*(8), 465-467. doi:10.3928/01484834-20090518-07

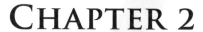

CHAPTER 2
SIMULATIONS: EDUCATION AND ETHICS
Sharon I. Decker, PhD, RN, ANEF, FAAN

"To know how to suggest is the
great art of teaching."

—Henri Frederic Amiel

THE DILEMMA

Kohn, Corrigan and Donaldson (1999) write that "it is simply not acceptable for patients to be harmed by the same health care system that is supposed to offer healing and comfort" (p. 3). The reality, however, is that the demand on health care providers has become more complex with the advancement of technology, the increasing complexity of patient care situations, the need for rapid decision-making despite conflicting or incomplete information, and increasing interdependence among members of the health care team (Hamman, 2004; Institute of Medicine [IOM], 2011; Long, 2004). Such realities demand a transformation in the educational process requiring changes in teaching, learning, and assessment strategies. The changes are mandatory to enhance learners' ability to develop the clinical reasoning and judgment required to provide safe effective patient care (Benner, Sutphen, Leonard, & Day,2009; IOM, 2011). As expressed by Thibault (2010), "We will not have robust, sustained health care reform unless we have a health professional workforce that is prepared to work in and lead the future system" (p. 6).

Patient safety is a major societal issue and is receiving attention from federal commissions, accreditation organizations, health care agencies, and consumer advocacy groups. The importance of the patient safety issue in health care is validated by multiple studies, and major causes of safety concerns have been identified. The cause of inadvertent harm to patients has been associated with ineffective communication between health care providers and inadequate orientation (Leonard, Graham, & Bonacum, 2004). For example, inadequate orientation of health care providers was identified as the underlying cause of 87 percent of deaths related to mechanical ventilation, and communication breakdown between health care providers accounts for 76 percent of deaths in such situations (Joint Commission on the Accreditation of Health Care Organizations [JCAHO], 2002). Additionally, ineffective communication among health care professionals was identified as the root cause of over 70 percent of sentinel events (JCAHO, 2005). The importance of patient safety was emphasized in the Joint Commission's patient safety goals (2011) which stressed the importance of interprofessional teamwork behaviors and communication to prevent medical errors.

As a member of the health care team, each individual is expected to promote safe, quality patient care through interprofessional collaboration, communication, and coordination. Research has demonstrated working together as an interprofessional team decreases costs, promotes patient satisfaction and safety, as well as improves the job satisfaction of health care providers (Allen, Penn, & Nora, 2006; Josiah Macy Jr. Foundation, 2010). The Lancet Commissions (Frenk et al., 2010) reported that the education of health care professionals "has not kept pace" with the challenge initiated by rapid demographic changes, new infections and diseases, changes in technology, and modifications in the health care delivery system (p. 5). Knettel (2011) stressed to remain cost competitive and improve quality and effectiveness the health care system "must make interprofessional collaborative practice a fundamental characteristic" (p. 2). Yet, Frenk and colleagues stated the educational issues being confronted by academic settings are systemic and relate to outdated, static curricula, poor teamwork, and the "tendency of various professionals to act in isolation" (p. 5).

Multiple accrediting agencies for health care professionals have written standards addressing the competency to function as a member of an interprofessional team. Professional organizations have presented position statements regarding interprofessional education and provided agreed-upon interprofessional competencies (Interprofessional Education Collaborative Expert Panel [IPEC], 2011). Among the strategies suggested to assist educators in transforming the educational process and assisting future health professionals in developing their intra-disciplinary and interprofessional competencies are simulation-based educational experiences to include the use of advanced patient simulators, standardized patients, haptic devices, virtual reality, and hybrid simulations (IOM 2011; IPEC; Koerner, 2003; Ziv, Wolpe, Small, & Glick, 2003).

ETHICAL CONSIDERATIONS

The identified societal issues of patient safety and the challenge to promote learning and competency through increased use of simulation require educators to consider the ethical considerations or dilemma of integrating simulation as an educational strategy in the teaching, learning, and evaluation process. Possible questions to consider are presented in Table 2-1.

Table 2-1 Thoughtful Questions to Consider
1. Would the inequity in social justice be minimized if health care students and practitioners were prepared and competencies validated through simulation?
2. Would the inequity in social justice be decreased if simulation were used to promote and validate interprofessional teamwork?
3. When informed consent is attained for a procedure, should a patient be provided with the qualifications of the individual performing the procedure? Is the principle of autonomy violated when informed consents do not provide full disclosure of all pertinent information?
4. What is the responsibility of faculty related to the use of simulation in the educational process, in light of research that validates that simulation promotes student learning while promoting a humanistic outlook toward patients?
5. Would learning through simulation prior to patient contact promote the competence of health care providers and thereby decrease the overuse of services?

Table 2-1 Thoughtful Questions to Consider - con't.
6. Does simulation provide a valid and reliable method to evaluate a student's and/or practitioner's competence and, if so, what is the obligation related to incorporating this technique into the evaluation process?
7. Is the act of not integrating simulation into the educational process of the health care student a form of neglect and, if so, could this cause an ethos of distrust (with both students and patients) and compromise the purpose of professional relationships?
8. Are educators demonstrating compassion when they allow health care students and practitioners to "practice" procedures on clients instead of providing simulated experiences?
9. In the future, will students and practitioners be required to demonstrate specific competencies in a simulated environment prior to engaging in actual patient care? In the future, will simulation play a role in licensure examinations and assessments for certification?
10. In the future, will simulation play a role in licensure examinations and assessments for certification?

THE PRINCIPLE OF JUSTICE

Justice as defined by Beauchamp and Childress (2001) is fairness or the "appropriate treatment in light of what is due or owed to persons" (p. 226). Social justice according to Beauchamp and Childress requires individuals to share equally in the benefits and risks of medical innovations, research, and practitioner training. Ziv and colleagues (2003) acknowledge that some citizens may be bearing a disproportionate amount of the benefits and risks related to practitioner training. Therefore, since research has demonstrated simulation (a) actively engages students in the learning process (Dillard et al., 2009; Lasater, 2007), (b) promotes clinical judgment (Kaddoura, 2010; Rhodes & Curran, 2005), and (c) facilitates the retention of knowledge specifically related to performing procedures (Jeffries, 2007; McGaghie, 2008), should educators ask, "Would the inequity in social justice be minimized if health care students are prepared and competencies validated through simulation prior to providing patient care?"

Kohn and colleagues (1999) identify the need to enhance teamwork within the health professions in an effort to promote mutual commitment and patient safety. Studies (Guise et al., 2010; Robertson et al., 2010; Shapiro et al., 2004) demonstrate an improvement in teamwork knowledge, communication skills, and team performance through simulation-based education. Therefore, another question to be considered is, "Would the inequity in social justice be decreased if simulation were used to promote and validate interprofessional teamwork?"

The Principle of Autonomy

Autonomy includes respect and acknowledges an individual's decision-making rights. Beauchamp and Childress (2001) state, "respect for autonomy is not a mere ideal in health care; it is a professional obligation" (p. 63). Autonomous choice, according to Beauchamp and Childress, "is a right, not a duty of patients" (p. 63). A question to discuss is, "Would the principle of autonomy be violated when informed consents do not provide full disclosure of all pertinent information?" Beauchamp and Childress also stress that "one gives an informed consent to an intervention if (and perhaps only if) one is competent to act, receives a thorough disclosure, comprehends the disclosure, acts voluntarily, and consents to the interventions" (p. 79). Therefore, should educators ask, "When informed consent is obtained for a procedure, should a patient be provided with the qualifications of the individual performing the procedure?" For example, should patients be told if a student is performing a venipuncture for the first time?

One could argue that patients admitted to teaching hospitals are generally aware that residents, interns, nursing and allied health students will be providing direct care. Yet a study by Cohen and colleagues (1987) revealed that only 37.5 percent of teaching hospitals that responded to the research survey specifically informed patients that students would be participating in their care. In addition, when many of these patients were questioned, they could not distinguish between a student and a health care professional.

The principle of autonomy related to students needs to be addressed when considering the use of simulation as a learning, teaching, and evaluation strategy. Ziv et al. (2003) emphasize that when student autonomy is respected, it leads to better educated students who develop a more humanistic outlook toward patients. Simulation can be used to identify (Morgan, Cleave-Hogg, DeSousa, &Tarshis, 2003; Rhodes & Curran, 2005) and support the learning needs of the student (Ziv et al.) and to promote the student's feelings of self-confidence (Bearnson & Wiker, 2005; Jeffries & Rizzolo, 2005; Smith & Roehrs, 2009). Therefore, a question to consider is if research validates simulation and promotes student learning while promoting a humanistic outlook toward patients, should nurse educators be questioning the responsibility of faculty related to the use of simulation in the educational process?

The Principle of Beneficence

As defined by Beauchamp and Childress (2001), beneficence "refers to an action done to benefit others; benevolence refers to the character trait or virtues of being disposed to act for the benefit of others (the capacity for promoting and achieving good); and principle of beneficence refers to a moral obligation to act for the benefit of others" (p. 166). Beneficence suggests that unwarranted care and the overuse of services should be prevented during patient care. Therefore, a question to be considered is, "Would learning through simulation prior to patient contact promote the competency of the health care providers and thereby decrease the overuse of services?" Another dilemma posed by Carlson (2011) is "What obligation is there to ensure that all providers, regardless of their location, have access to simulation training not only so they as providers are competent but also so the patient population they serve receives competent care?" (p. 12).

THE PRINCIPLE OF NONMALEFICENCE

According to the principle of nonmaleficence, an individual ought not to inflict harm, including emotional, physical, and financial injury (Beauchamp & Childress, 2001). Yet, according to Smith and Crawford (2003), many avoidable errors in health care continue to be correlated to inaccessible data and the inability of newly licensed registered nurses to make clinical decisions based on data obtained from physical assessments and diagnostic tests. Furthermore, The Code of Ethics for Nurses (American Nurses Association, 2001) stresses, "Nurse Educators have a responsibility to ensure that basic competencies are achieved ... prior to entry of an individual into practice" (p. 13). Yet, studies indicate nursing students are graduating without the appropriate competencies to practice in the work setting (Berkow & Virkstis, 2008; Hickey, 2009). Among the deficiencies are competencies related to interpretation of assessment data, recognition of changes in patient status, and medication administrative skills. Therefore, a question that could be debated is, "Does simulation provide a valid and reliable method to evaluate a student's competency and, if so, what is the educator's obligation related to incorporating this technique into the evaluation process?" For example, Ziv, Small, and Wolpe (2000) stress that the use of patient simulators can provide consistent learning and evaluation of experience, to include atypical patterns, rare diseases, critical incidents, near misses, and crises. These experts stress that educators have "an ethical obligation to make all efforts to expose a health professional to clinical challenges that can be reasonably well simulated prior to allowing them to encounter and be responsible for similar real-life challenges" (p. 492). A question posed by Carlson (2011) related to the principle of nonmaleficenceis, "Is it ethical for some providers to receive simulation-based competency training and other providers not to be given the opportunity?" (p. 12).

THE PRINCIPLE OF VERACITY

Veracity is defined by Beauchamp and Childress (2001) as not intentionally deceiving or misleading a patient. Pellegrino and Thomasma (1993) stress "trust and self-effacement can be, and must be, indispensable traits of the authentic professional" (p. 158). The virtue of trust is acknowledged as central and indispensable to the nurse-patient (or faculty-student) relationship. Peter and Morgan (2001) stress that trust is an obligation, not a privilege, and that without trust, the healing or helping goal cannot be attained. Therefore, a question to be addressed could be, "Is the act of not integrating simulation into the education of the health care students a form of neglect, and if so, could this cause an ethos of distrust (with both students and patients) and compromise the purpose of professional relationships?"

THE PRINCIPLE OF COMPASSION

Compassion is discussed by Pellegrino and Thomasma (1993) as an essential virtue in health care delivery. The authors stress that "compassion and competence go hand in hand as necessary and mutually reinforcing virtues"; this is further emphasized by the statement, "nothing is more inconsistent with compassion than the well-meaning, empathetic, but incompetent clinician" (p. 83). Therefore, a question that could be considered is, "Are nurse educators and other health care professionals demonstrating compassion when they allow students to perform procedures for the first time on clients instead of first providing students with simulated experiences?"

SUMMARY

As technology advances, computerized simulations will become more realistic and provide students and health care professionals opportunities to learn and remain proficient in most procedures without endangering patient safety. Final questions that need to be addressed include "What is the health care educator's responsibility in providing simulation-based education as it related to patient safety?" and "In the future, will students be required to demonstrate specific competencies prior to engaging in actual patient care?" Educators are required to ensure patient safety while providing educational opportunities for students to develop the competency needed to provide patient care. Therefore, educators have the responsibility to advocate in the interest of both the student and the patient while promoting change in the culture of nursing education.

References

Allen, D. D., Penn, M. A., Nora, L. M. (2006). Interdisciplinary healthcare education: Fact of fiction? *American Journal of Pharmaceutical Education, 70*(2), 1-2.

American Nurses Association. (2001). *Code of ethics for nurses with interpretive standards.* Washington, DC: American Nurses Publishing.

Bearnson, C. S., & Wiker, K. M. (2005). Human patient simulators: A new face in baccalaureate nursing education at Brigham Young University. *Journal of Nursing Education, 44*(9), 421-425.

Beauchamp, T. L., & Childress, J. F. (2001). *Principles of biomedical ethics* (3rd ed.). Washington, DC: Oxford University Press.

Benner, P., Sutphen, M., Leonard, V., & Day, L. (2009). *Educating nurses: A call for radical transformation.* San Francisco, CA: Jossey-Bass.

Berkow, J. K., & Virkstis, K. (2008). Assessing new graduate nurse performance. J*ournal of Nursing Administration, 32*, 509-523.

Carlson, E. (2011). Ethical consideration surrounding simulation-based competency training., *Journal of Illinois Nursing, 109*(3), 11- 14.

Cohen, D. L., McCullough, L. B., Kessel, R. W., Apostolides, A. Y., Alden, E. R., & Heiderich, K. L. (1987). Informed consent policies governing medical students' interaction with patients. *Journal of Medical Education, 62*(10), 789-798.

Dillard, N., Sideras, S., Ryan, M., Carlton, K. H., Lasater, K., & Siktberg, L. (2009). A collaborative project to apply and evaluate the clinical judgment model through simulation. *Nursing Education Perspectives, 30*(2), 99-104.

Frenk, J., Chen, L., Bhutta, Z.A., Cohen, J., Crisp, N., Evans, T., ... Zurayk, H. (2010). Health professionals for a new century: transforming education to strengthen health systems in an interdependent world. *Lancet, 376*, 1923–1958.

Guise, J. M., Lowe, N. K., Deering, S., Lewis, P. O., O'Haire, C., Irwin, L. K., . . . Kanki, B. G. (2010). Mobile in situ obstetric emergency simulation and teamwork training to improve maternal-fetal safety in hospitals. *The Joint Commission Journal on Quality and Patient Safety, 36*(10), 443-453.

Hamman, W. R. (2004, October). The complexity of team training: What we have learned from aviation and its applications to medicine. *Quality & Safety in Health Care, 13* (Suppl. 1), i72-i79.

Institute of Medicine. (2011). T*he future of nursing leading change, advancing health*. Washington, DC: The National Academies Press.

Interprofessional Education Collaborative Expert Panel. (2011). *Core competencies for interprofessional collaborative practice: Report of an expert panel*. Washington, DC: Interprofessional Education Collaborative.

Jeffries, P., & Rizzolo, M. A. (2005, June). *NLN/Laerdal simulation study: Phase III, part 2*. Paper presented at the Study Project Coordinators Meeting, San Antonio, TX.

Jeffries, P. R. (Ed.). (2007). *Simulations in nursing education: From conceptualization to evaluation*. New York, NY: The National League for Nursing.

The Joint Commission. (2011). Critical access hospitals: 2011 national patient safety goals. In *www.jointcommission.org*. Retrieved July 5, 2012 from http://www. jointcommission.org/assets/1/6/2011_NPSGs_CAH.pdf.

Joint Commission on Accreditation of Healthcare Organizations. (2002, February 26). Sentinel event alert (Issue 25). In www.jointcommission.org. Retrieved July 5, 2012, from http://www.jointcommission.org/ SentinelEvents/SentinelEventAlert/sea_25.htm

Joint Commission on Accreditation of Healthcare Organizations. (2005). National patient safety goals. In www.jointcommission.org. Retrieved July 5, 2012, from http://www.jointcommission.org/PatientSafety/ NationalPatientSafetyGoals.

Josiah Macy Jr. Foundation. (2010). Preparing health professional for a changing healthcare system. In *www.macyfoundation.org*. Retrieved July 5, 2012, from www.macyfoundation.org.

Kaddoura, M. A. (2010). New graduate nurses' perceptions of the effects of clinical simulation on the critical thinking, learning, and confidence. *The Journal of Continuing Education in Nursing, 41*(11), 506-516.

Knettel, A. (2011). Making the business case for interprofessional education and training. *In Association of Academic Health Centers.* Retrieved July 5, 2012 from http://www.aahcdc.org/Resources/ReportsAndPublications/IssueBriefs/View/tabid/79/ArticleId/103/The-Business-Case-for-Academic-Health-Centers-Addressing-Environmental-Social-and-Behavioral-Determi.aspx.

Koerner, J. G. (2003). The virtues of the virtual world: Enhancing the technology/knowledge professional interface for life-long learning. Nursing *Administration Quarterly, 27*(1), 9-17.

Kohn, L., Corrigan, J., & Donaldson, M. (Eds.). (1999). *To err is human: Building a safer health system.* Washington, DC: National Academy of Science.

Lasater, K. (2007). High-fidelity simulation and the development of clinical judgment: Students' experiences. *Journal of Nursing Education, 46*(6), 269-275.

Leonard, M., Graham, S., & Bonacum, D. (2004). The human factor: The critical importance of effective teamwork and communication in providing safe care. *Quality & Safety in Health Care, 13* (Suppl. 1), i85-i90.

McGaghie, W. C. (2008). Research opportunities in simulation-based medical education using deliberate practice. *Academic Emergency Medicine, 15*(11), 995-1001.

Morgan, P. J., Cleave-Hogg, D., DeSousa, S., & Tarshis, J. (2003). Identification of gaps in the achievement of undergraduate anesthesia educational objectives using high-fidelity patient simulation. *Anesthesia & Analgesia, 97*, 1690-1694.

Pellegrino, E. D., & Thomasma, D. C. (1993). *The virtues in medical practice.* New York, NY: Oxford University Press.

Peter, E., & Morgan, K. P. (2001). Exploration of a trust approach for nursing ethics. *Nursing Inquiry, 8*(1), 3-10.

Rhodes, M. L., & Curran, C. (2005). Use of the human patient simulator to teach clinical judgment skills in baccalaureate nursing programs. *Computers in Nursing, 23*(5), 256-262.

Robertson, B., Kaplan, B., Atallah, H., Higgins, M., Lewitt, M. J., & Ander, D. S. (2010). The use of simulation and a modified TeamSTEPPS curriculum for medical and nursing student team training. *Simulation in Healthcare, 5*(6), 332-337.

Shapiro, M. J., Morey, J. C., Small, S. D., Langford, V., Kayor, C. J., Jagminas, L., . . . Jay, G. D. (2004). Simulation based teamwork training for emergency department staff: Does it improve clinical team performance when added to an existing didactic teamwork curriculum? *Quality & Safety in Health Care, 13*(6), 417-421.

Smith, J., & Crawford, L. (2003). Report of findings from the practice and professional issues survey. *National Council of State Boards of Nursing Research Brief, 7.*

Smith, S. J., & Roehrs, C. J. (2009) High-fidelity simulation: Factors correlated with nursing student satisfaction and self-confidence. *Nursing Education Perspective, 30*(2), 74-78.

Thibault, G. E. (2010). President's statement. In *Josiah Macy Jr. Foundation. Preparing health professionals for a changing healthcare system.* Retrieved July 5, 2012 from www. macyfoundation.org

Ziv, A., Wolpe, P. R., Small, S. D., & Glick, S. (2003). Simulation-based medical education: An ethical imperative. *Academic Medicine, 78*(8), 783-788.

CHAPTER 3

THEORETICAL FRAMEWORK FOR SIMULATION DESIGN

Pamela R. Jeffries, PhD, RN, FAAN, ANEF
Kristen J. Rogers, MSN, RN

"If you have knowledge,
let others light their candles at it"

—Margaret Fuller

Introduction

When simulation is conducted without benefit of an organizing framework, influencing variables cannot be studied in a consistent way and educators have difficulty determining the effectiveness of various practices. It prevents scholars from conducting research in an organized, systemic fashion and influencing factors become elusive, as does the effectiveness of various parts. To adequately assess learner outcomes a conceptual framework that specifies relevant variables and their relationships is critical. Nurse educators as well as leaders in medical education have identified the need for a consistent and empirically supported model to guide simulation design and implementation and to assess learner outcomes when using simulations (Cioffi, 2001; Hotchkiss, Biddle, & Fallard, 2002). In response to this need, the National League for Nursing set out to develop and test a simulation design framework.

The framework proposed here was originally developed based on insights gained from the theoretical and empirical literature related to simulations in nursing, medicine, and other health care disciplines, as well as non-health care disciplines. It was developed for and initially tested through the National League for Nursing/Laerdal simulation study (Jeffries, 2005) and is named NLN/Jeffries Simulation Framework (National League for Nursing [NLN], 2012). Although it has been several years since its development, components of the simulation framework have been used and tested by various educational researchers, including master's and doctoral students. These researchers have found the NLN/Jeffries Simulation Framework serves an important purpose with very minor edits to correlate with the terms used today in simulation.

The NLN/Jeffries Simulation Framework has five conceptual components (Figure 1), each of which is operationalized through a number of variables. The five concepts originally included (a) teacher factors (now facilitator), (b) students factors (now participant), (c) educational practices that need to be incorporated into the instruction, (d) simulation design characteristics, and (e) expected student outcomes. In 2011, the International Nursing Association of Clinical Simulations and Learning (INACSL) developed a research task force to review the simulation framework and its constructs to consider if the framework can move to a theory. The project reviewed and reined the five major concepts of the framework with the aim to (a) define and refine the concepts, (b) evaluate existing research/literature, (c) suggest appropriate revisions, (d) suggest testable hypotheses for future research, and (e) advance the science of nursing simulation. Twenty expert nurse researchers/educators (including two nurse theorists) facilitated by Dr. Patty Ravert, primary investigator, PI of the project, formed five teams along the lines of the major framework concepts. From this work, two teams recommended changing the titles of their concepts — student to participant and teacher to facilitator. The results and recommendations were presented in 2012 at the International Nursing Simulation Learning Resource Center Conference.

During the presentations the conference participants were queried for confirmation of recommendations and other points to be further evaluated by the teams. Each of the components of the framework is further discussed in the following sections.

NLN/Jeffries Simulation Framework

All instructional strategies, including simulations, should be based on what is known about learning and cognition (Bednar, Cunningham, Duffy, & Perry, 1995), and educators often use an eclectic approach that selects principles and techniques from a variety of theoretical perspectives. For example, collaborative educational learning tools have been based upon behavioral, cognitive information processing, humanistic, and socio-cultural theories. Computer-based teaching strategies have drawn upon adult learning, constructivist, and cognitive learning theories.

The use of simulations in education has most often been grounded in theories that focus on learner-centered practices, constructivism, and socio-cultural collaboration between individuals with different socio-cultural backgrounds. Concepts of learning and cognition (Cunningham, 1996) relevant in designing and using simulations include mind as computer, mind as brain, and mind as rhizome, that is, providing for an infinite number of connections within and without the social cultural milieu. These metaphors, respectively, point to a view of learning as information processing that is (a) a cognitive skill, (b) experiential growth and pattern recognition, and (c) a socio-cultural dialogue. When learning is viewed as information processing, instruction is focused on providing efficient communication of information and emphasis is on remembering. When learning is viewed as experiential growth, instruction focuses on experiences and activities that promote the development of cognitive networks and understanding. Finally, when learning is viewed as a socio-cultural dialogue, instruction provides opportunities for embedding learning in realistic tasks that lead learners toward participation in a community of practice. Simulations are relevant to each of these perspectives. We must consider the socio-cultural aspects within a simulation environment to provide the real-world dialogue and environment.

Simulation in Nursing Education Framework Components

The NLN/Jeffries Simulation Framework has five different components that will be described here. Examples of the framework component will be provided and evidence cited for the component when available.

The Facilitator

The facilitator is essential to the success of any learning experience. In clinical education, the teacher facilitates, guides, critiques, and evaluates student performance (Ard, Rogers, & Vinten, 2008). However, unlike many traditional classrooms that are teacher-centered, simulations are student-centered, with the educator playing the roles of facilitator and evaluator.

As a facilitator, the educator may provide support and encouragement to the learner throughout the simulation, asking questions, proposing "what if" situations, and guiding the debriefing at the conclusion of the experience. The facilitator should ask thought provoking questions that result in students thinking beyond the obvious (Gaberson & Oermann, 2010). As an evaluator, the educator typically serves strictly as an observer. In simulated clinical experience, students suggest that effective instructors should serve as partners and offer them support through decision-making (Parsh, 2010).

Facilitators must feel comfortable with and be prepared for the simulations they are using, and they may require assistance with designing the simulation, using the technology, setting up equipment for the activity, and fulfilling the roles of the facilitator and evaluator. In a faculty development workshop where faculty members were immersed in a simulation experience, Johnson, Zeric, and Theis (1999) reported that faculty experienced feelings similar to those of students. This activity enabled faculty to identify with students' anxiety and discomforts while participating in this new experience. As part of the simulation framework, selected demographics, such as years of experience, age of the facilitator, and clinical expertise, are believed to be associated with the teacher's role, experience, comfort, and overall use of simulations. Reese (2010) analyzed the educator role in simulations by exploring the classroom and clinical teacher effectiveness attributes and characteristics. From her research, she developed the the the Student Perception of Effective Teaching in Clinical Simulation (SPETCS), a unique 33-item survey instrument developed to measure teaching behaviors in simulation contexts using a five-point Likert scale. The measure contains two separate response scales, Extent and Importance. The Extent scale measures participants' perception of the extent to which the educator used a particular teaching strategy during the simulation, and the Importance scale measures perception of the degree of importance of the teaching strategy toward meeting simulation learning outcomes. In Reese's findings, the top five highest item measures pertaining to teacher effectiveness facilitating during simulations included (a) useful feedback from instructor; (b) improved ability of the participant to care for a patient with similar problems; (c) development of critical thinking skills in simulations; (d) perception that debriefing supported clinical reasoning; and (e) fidelity of the simulation. Her work noted the importance of teacher contributions to making a simulation successful and impactful to the learner.

Further research is needed in this area to explore relationships between selected teacher characteristics and the use of simulations in nursing education.

The Participant

Although simulation experiences differ, participants generally are expected to be responsible for their own learning, meaning they need to be self-directed and motivated. Learners are more likely to fulfill this responsibility if they know the ground rules for the activity. Such rules encourage and support learning, acknowledge that mistakes are part of the process, and minimize competition, which, although a common human motivator, often is detrimental to learning because it may increase anxiety and stress. The ground rules also specify the roles various learners will play during the simulation. If the simulation involves group role-playing, the educator should inform participants about the specific role each is to play. Roles vary with the simulation, but the most common are patient, nurse, family member, another health care professional, or an unlicensed assistive staff member. In addition, participants might also play the role of an observer, recorder, or documenter. Simulation participants may rotate through various roles as the simulation is experienced and they should discuss each role during the debriefing that follows the experiences. Participants should be immersed only in the roles that pertain to their scope of practice or as family members or other tactile-type roles. Immersing the learner in the role of the physician would be beyond the learner's scope of practice and could cause a very negative learning experience for all.

Cioffi (2001) discussed two types of participant roles, response-based and process-based, that can be played during a simulation experience. In a response-based role, the learner is not an active participant and has no control over the material presented. An example of this would be assigning a participant the role of an observer during the simulation experience. In this role, the student can be part of the simulation but is instructed not to talk, make decisions, or problem solve during the simulation. In the process-based method, the learner is an active participant, making decisions on what information to assess or seek from written resources, the patient, and/or family, as well as the sequence and time to seek important information about the client. Examples of this format are patient role-plays, vignettes, and other simulator/simulation activities.

Participants also engage in activities designed to judge their progress towards attaining learning outcomes. One such participant activity is self-evaluation while viewing a videotape of their performance and using the same critical skills checklist that was used by the faculty during their "live" patient scenario (Gibbons et al., 2002). Boet et al. (2011) had students participate in a self-debriefing session while viewing their participation in a high-fidelity simulation on crisis management skills. This technique resulted in an improvement in students' knowledge base, as evidenced through improved post-test results.

As with the educator concept in the simulation model, the participant concept also encompasses variables that may affect the individual's simulation experience, performance, and overall learning outcomes when being involved in a simulation activity. For example, these characteristics might include the participant's age and any experience in nursing care prior to their formal education. In a qualitative study conducted by McCurry and Martins (2010), the participants that were Millennial learners preferred interactive activities and activities that involved teamwork. More research is needed to explore these variables and the impact they have on students and learning outcomes

EDUCATIONAL PRACTICES IN SIMULATION

The educational practices component of the simulation framework addresses the features of active learning, feedback, diverse learning styles, and collaboration. These features need to be considered when designing a simulation to improve student performance and satisfaction with their learning (Chickering & Gamson, 1987).

Active learning

According to Reilly and Oermann (1990), the adult learner will lose interest in an educational experience without active involvement; this engagement in the learning process is critical when designing and using simulations. Active engagement has been shown to enhance students' critical thinking skills (Billings & Halstead, 2011), and it also provides the educator an opportunity to assess the learner's problem solving and decision-making skills within the context of the simulation experience. Students have also indicated that active learning in a simulation is important to their learning and knowledge retention (Swenty & Eggleston, 2011).

Feedback

Feedback to learners is important to incorporate into any simulation, but whether that feedback should occur during or after the simulation or both needs to be considered carefully. The facilitator also needs to decide on the frequency of feedback. Although extensive feedback might be assumed to be helpful, it is important to remember that a simulation should create a safe environment for the learner where mistakes can be made (Henneman & Cunningham, 2005) and where excessive feedback may not be appropriate. If feedback is provided during a simulation, it is important to be careful not to interfere with the learning process. Instead the learner should be allowed to make a decision, take action, and reflect on that action before feedback is given. Typically, feedback should be given after the simulated experience so the learner has the opportunity to perform and function in the professional role, making decisions and problem solving in the learning situation designed. If educators provide feedback during the simulation, the learner may become dependent upon the instructor for "next steps" or gestures of what to do next.

Diverse Learning Styles

According to Dunn and Griggs (1998), understanding that students come to a learning experience with diverse learning styles can help educators optimize learning. In one study on learning styles and student satisfaction with high-fidelity simulation, Fountain and Alfred (2009) showed that student learning styles of solitary learning and social learning were satisfied with high-fidelity simulation.

Since students might be visual, auditory, tactile, or kinesthetic learners, educators need to incorporate activities into simulations that meet the needs of all learning styles. Fortunately, it is quite easy to do this when designing a simulation, but the degree of emphasis on a learning style will vary depending on the goals and complexity of the simulation.

In the NLN/Laerdal simulation project (Jeffries, 2007) strategies were incorporated for all four learning styles. For visual learners, the room was set up to reflect a "real-life" client room; the clock was set to the appropriate time for the beginning of the day shift (seven o'clock in the morning) and the date was posted on the wall. The auditory learner was accommodated by alarms sounding when the heart rate was too high and other types of beeps and sounds that are normally found in the hospital environment, as well as through verbal sounds of SimMan™ programming of verbal responses and through interacting with a student-role-played "family member." The tactile learning style was incorporated though the use of SimMan because the learner could auscultate lung, bowel, and heart sounds, palpate pulses, and obtain blood pressure readings. Finally, in the client's room, there were dressing supplies, an inspiratory spirometer, and medications, which appealed to the kinesthetic learners because they could actually handle equipment for implementing care.

Student-Faculty Feedback

According to Billings and Halstead (2011), the student-faculty relationship can influence the learning experience. To have a positive impact, the relationship must be collaborative and provide an arena for the exchange of information. This will foster a climate of mutual respect in which the learner feels comfortable asking questions that enhance learning. In developing the simulation, the educator needs to aim for this type of atmosphere. Constructive feedback provided by the faculty after the simulation is essential to foster learning. Gaberson and Oermann (2010) found that feedback about performance should be specific, including information about any problems with decision-making. For the feedback to be effective it should be given to the student at the time of learning or immediately after the experience. Additionally, the feedback needs to be diagnostic and the teacher should provide guidance for the student in how to improve performance. The educator also needs to obtain feedback from the learner about the simulation experience that will help the educator refine the experience. Also, feedback provides an opportunity to address concerns expressed by the learner and promotes active learner involvement in the learning process.

High Expectations

It has been said that when people are expected to do well and they are given the guidance and support needed to succeed, they do succeed. This principle is as relevant for students in a simulation learning experience as it is in other aspects of life. Learners should set personal learning goals with faculty members and seek advice on how to achieve those goals. When both facilitators and participants have high expectations for the simulation experience and the outcomes, positive results most often are achieved. Vandrey and Whitman (2001) found that in a safe learning environment using simulations, nurses are able to expand their competency levels and feel empowered to achieve greater learning. At Georgetown University Hospital, critical care nurses participate in high-frequency, high-acuity simulations to enhance their ability to provide care to patients. These simulations have been evaluated as positive by the nurses and the instructors. Through these simulations, nurses have increased their confidence and identified opportunities for improvement (Rauen, 2004).

SIMULATION AND DESIGN FEATURES

Design characteristics should incorporate the following five features: objectives, fidelity, problem solving, student support, and reflective thinking (debriefing), all of which must be addressed when developing a simulation. The educator needs to define the features in relation to the simulation purpose and determine the level of inclusion of each feature. The level of inclusion will depend upon the intended outcomes of the simulation.

Objectives/Information

According to Reilly and Oermann (1990), objectives are the tools that guide learning, and they are essential when using simulations. The objectives of the simulation must reflect the intended outcome of the experience, specify expected learner behaviors, and include sufficient detail to allow the learner to participate in the simulation effectively.

In the NLN/Laerdal simulation research project (Jeffries, 2007), prior to beginning each experience, learners were provided with the purpose and objectives of the simulation. The simulation facilitator read a scripted orientation to the learners that provided a brief overview of the different parts of the simulation experience, the timeframes, students' roles, and a review of the objectives. The objectives were used at the beginning of the simulation to provide direction to the student learners as they were preparing for the experience. After the simulation, reference to the objectives can be included in the debriefing, with learners explaining how they met the objectives and instructors validating the completion of the objectives.

Fidelity

Fidelity refers to the extent to which a simulation mimics reality; there are three levels of sophistication (Seropian, 2003 — high, moderate, and low. High-fidelity simulation incorporates a sophisticated computerized manikin that can mimic a real-life situation; for example, the manikin's chest rises and falls. In a moderate-fidelity simulation with the manikin, for example, the chest looks real and breath sounds can be heard, but the chest does not rise and fall. A low-fidelity simulation incorporates static tools (Long, 2005), for example, a manikin with no extra features such as breath and heart sounds, voice, or any interactive features.

If the purpose of the simulation is skill attainment, for example, IM injection, then a low-fidelity simulation such as an injection pad and a syringe is sufficient. If the purpose of the simulation is introducing students to assessment skills, then a moderate-fidelity simulation can provide students with feedback such as heart and lung sounds (Campbell, 2010). If the purpose of the experience is to enhance the students' critical thinking skills in caring for clients with end-stage kidney disease, a high-fidelity simulation would provide a "close-to-life" situation that allows for patient-nurse communication and exhibition of appropriate signs and symptoms. In developing a high-fidelity simulation, the real-life situation should be replicated as closely as possible (Medley & Horne, 2005).

There are several researchers that categorize realism into different categories. For example, Beaubian and Baker (2004) discuss three dimensions of realism which include the (a) equipment, (b) environment, and (c) psychological. Their first dimension, equipment fidelity, concerns the degree to which the simulator duplicates the appearance and feel of the real system. For example, a simulator that realistically mimics a human being that has cardiac, respiratory, and bowel sounds in addition to physiological modeling as demonstrated when a medication is given and the simulator acts accordingly to the way the drug is intended, could be described as high in equipment fidelity. Their second dimension, environment fidelity, concerns the extent to which the simulator duplicates motion cues, visual cues, and other sensory information from the task environment. For example, when caring for a deteriorating patient in a critical care simulated area, the simulation could be defined as high (or low) on environment fidelity, depending on whether the motion and cues were turned on (or off) and present; for example, alarms sounding on the monitor, the intravenous pump beeping, and the heart rate on the monitor demonstrating an erratic and rapid pattern, with all demonstrating environment fidelity. Their third dimension, psychological fidelity, concerns the degree to which the participant perceives the simulation to be a believable surrogate for the trained task. Alternatively, it could be defined as the match between the participant's performance in the simulator and the real world. For example, a high-fidelity patient simulator could be defined as high in psychological fidelity if the participants temporarily suspend disbelief and interact much as they would in the real world.

Lauken (1995) and Goffman (1974) describe reality in three other ways of thinking: phenomenal, which is represented by emotions, self-awareness, and beliefs; the physical; and semantical (does the information conceptually and theoretically make sense). Simulations provide an opportunity for learners to experience the social phenomena of experiencing reality through different elements designed in the scenario.

Goffman (1974) argues that the concept of simulations is a social practice. He discusses how simulations are created as a primary frame that are basic cognitive structures guiding the representation of reality. In other words, the primary frame provides a primary guide on how humans believe what is going on in the simulation scenario. The primary frame will help the participant to make sense of the simulation and activities. However, there are what Goffman calls "modulations" that account for the learner's world orientation of the scenario. These modulations can be experiences brought into the scenario such as anxiety, feelings of being exposed, and other types of emotions that can create "negative learning." The researchers believe the modulations need to be addressed to promote positive learning.

Problem Solving

Problem solving is related to the level of complexity of the simulation, which in turn needs to be based on the knowledge and skill level of the learners. The educator needs to reflect on the purpose of the experience and the learner's abilities when determining the level of complexity. A complex simulation should be at a level that is challenging to the learner but attainable. If the level is unattainable, the simulation will not be an effective learning experience for the learner. It is important not to overload the learner with too much information just because the simulator has a variety of options (Rauen, 2001); although it is important to try to mimic a real-life situation. In a complex simulation, the educator wants to provide the learner an opportunity to prioritize nursing assessments, provide care based on the assessments, and then be able to perform a self-evaluation.

Participant Support and Cues

The support feature focuses on the assistance provided to the participant. In creating the simulation, the educator needs to determine how and when support and assistance will be provided by the facilitator, a cue from another individual involved in the simulation, a lab report, a phone call, or another type of cueing mechanism. Assistance should be in the form of cues that offer enough information for the learner to continue with the simulation but do not interfere with his/her independent problem solving. For example, if the student is performing a head-to-toe assessment and the patient begins to experience chest tightness, the student may be so focused on the assessment that she ignores the complaint of chest tightness. The educator can provide cues through programming the patient simulator to verbalize the pain or instructing the "family" ahead of time to ask if the nurse could do something about the patient's pain if necessary, as it is not like him to complain. Cues like this alert the nurse to the patient's pain and, hopefully, will direct the assessments and attention to this patient problem.

Reflective thinking

According to the International Nursing Association for Clinical Simulation and Learning (INACSL), reflective thinking should be incorporated into all simulated experiences. According to Shinnick, Woo, Horwich, and Steadman (2011), the greatest knowledge gains occurred when students participated in a simulation followed by a debriefing session. The debriefing session allows for building of confidence. In a qualitative study on clinical simulation, students stated the following about debriefing: "I realized things I did not do well," "helped me to see the bigger picture," and "suggestions were helpful" (Courdeau, 2010). A debriefing session should occur immediately after the simulation is completed so the thoughts and feelings of the learner are not forgotten and do not get distorted over time.

The reflective thinking session needs to be guided by the facilitator so remarks focus on the learning outcomes and the application of learned concepts to practice (Rauen, 2001). The facilitator should have observed the simulation and be competent in the debriefing process. For the debriefing to be effective, the facilitator must create a supportive environment that fosters open communication and self-analysis (INACSL Board of Directors, 2011).

Discussion is often enhanced if the facilitator develops specific topics for discussion that are related to the objectives. For example, to prioritize nursing concerns for the client, the discussion focuses on constructive comments and learning instead of criticism (Medley & Horne, 2005). Table 1 lists the questions used during the reflective thinking session of the NLN/Laerdal simulation study (NLN, 2006). These questions evolved from the objectives of the simulation experience and helped the educator assess how well they had been met. The questions also helped the educator clarify any misperceptions, correct any errors that had been made, and emphasize correct, appropriate, and safe nursing care and decision-making.

OUTCOMES

The final component of the Simulation Model (Figure 1) is outcomes, such as knowledge gained, skills performed, participants' satisfaction, critical thinking, and self-confidence. This list of outcomes is only a few and not meant to be exhaustive. Today, there are many outcomes being assessed using simulations. For example, Reese, Jeffries, and Engum (2010) created an interprofessional simulation to measure outcomes of interdisciplinary communication and collaboration. Bambini, Washburn, and Perkins (2009) utilized simulation to measure the outcomes of communication, confidence, and clinical judgment. Ironside and Jeffries (2010) measured patient safety competencies in a simulation focused on care of multiple patients. Simulations have been incorporated into an introductory neonatal intensive care unit course for nurses as a method to improve patient safety and staff retention (Broussard, Myers, & Lemoine, 2009). Leonard, Shuhaibar, and Chen (2010) used high-fidelity simulations for role recognition and differentiation, adaptation to team environment, and professional solidarity. Bensfield, Olech, and Horsley (2012) utilized high-fidelity simulation in the final semester for summative evaluation. Through this simulation, students in need of remediation were identified. Individualized remediation plans were then created based on the students' simulation performance. Eggenberger, Keller, and Locsin (2010) explored the outcome of caring behaviors expressed within an emergent nursing situation using a high-fidelity simulator.

As noted, learning outcomes need to be established and discussed prior to the simulation. Additionally, the approaches and tools to be used to measure attainment of the objectives must be established in advance. Evaluating outcomes is essential to determine what learners have obtained and the overall effectiveness of the simulation experience (Kirkpatrick, DeWitt-Weaver, & Yeager, 2005). The nurse educator might want to ask questions such as the following to evaluate the simulation experience: Did it provide the type of experience desired by the instructor and students? Was it an effective use of faculty time and resources? Were there problems or concerns with the implementation phase of the simulation? Did the simulation produce the pre-established outcomes? What revisions are necessary? Are appropriate evaluation methods being used to assess the outcomes needed? Did the student learn the objectives outlined for the simulation? Did the simulation provide the learning outcomes expected for the learner?

SUMMARY

A framework that identifies significant components of simulations and the relationships among these components is a very useful guide to the design, implementation, and evaluation of simulation activities. Teaching and learning using simulations are complex, multi-faceted, and challenging. It is hoped that the use of the NLN/Jeffries Simulation

Framework described here will enhance the development, implementation, and evaluation of this exciting and innovative teaching-learning strategy in nursing education.

The NLN/Jeffries Simulation Framework

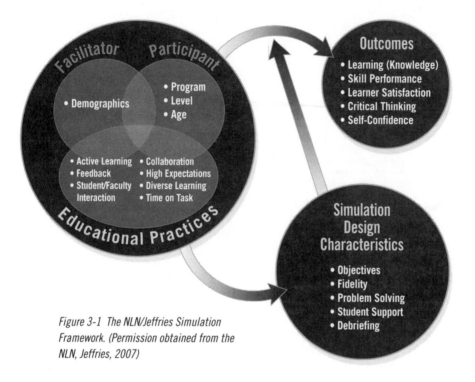

Figure 3-1 *The NLN/Jeffries Simulation Framework. (Permission obtained from the NLN, Jeffries, 2007)*

Table 3-1 Reflective Thinking Questions

1. How did you feel throughout the simulation experience?
2. Describe the objectives you were able to achieve.
3. Which ones were you unable to achieve (if any)?
4. Did you have the knowledge and skills to meet objectives?
5. Were you satisfied with your ability to work through the situation?
6. To Observer: Could the nurses have handled any aspects of the simulation differently?
7. If you were able to do this again, how could you have handled the situation differently?
8. What did the group do well?
9. What did the team think was the primary nursing diagnosis?
10. What were the key assessments and interventions?
11. Is there anything else you would like to discuss?

Table 3-2 Reflective Thinking Session Guidelines

1. The person who conducts the reflective thinking must observe the simulation.

2. Immediately after the simulation, the students are taken away from the bedside to a separate room for guided reflection.

3. The guided reflection session should last 20 minutes — 10 minutes for discussing content and 10 minutes for reflective thinking.

4. The facilitator doing the debriefing should correct and discuss any inappropriate actions that occurred, missed assessments, or interventions.

5. If time runs out and students still want to discuss the event, direct them to use reflective journaling and turn journals in to the instructor.

6. Give a five minute warning before the end of the simulation itself and before the end of the reflective thinking session.

REFERENCES

Ard, N., Rogers, K., & Vinten, S. (2008). Summary of the survey on clinical education in nursing. *Nursing Education Perspectives, 29*(4), 238-245.

Bambini, D., Washburn, J., & Perkins, R. (2009). Outcomes of clinical simulation for novice nursing students: Communication, confidence, clinical judgment. *Nursing Education Perspectives, 30*(2), 79-82.

Beaubien, J. M., & Baker, D. P. (2004). The use of simulation for training teamwork skills in health care: How low can you go? *Quality & Safety in Health Care, 13* (Suppl. 1), i51-i56.

Bednar, A., Cunningham, D. J., Duffy, T., & Perry, D. (1995). Theory in practice: How do we link? In G. Anglin (Ed.), *Instructional Technology: Past, present, and future* (pp. 100-112). Englewood, CO: Libraries Unlimited.

Bensfield, L. A., Olech, M. J., & Horsley, T. L. (2012). Simulation for high-stakes evaluation in nursing. *Nurse Educator, 37*(2), 71-74.

Billings, D., & Halstead, J. (2011). *Teaching in nursing: A guide for faculty* (4th ed.). Philadelphia, PA: W. B. Saunders.

Boet, S., Bould, M. D., Bruppacher, H. R., Desjardins, F., Chandra, D. B., & Naik, V. N. (2011). Looking in the mirror: Self-debrieing versus instructor debriefing for a simulated crises. *Critical Care Medicine, 39*(6), 1377-1381.

Broussard, L., Myers, R., & Lemoine, J. (2009). Preparing pediatric nurses: The role of simulation-based learning. *Issues in Comprehensive Pediatric Nursing, 32*, 4-15.

Campbell, S. H. (2010). Clinical simulation. In K. B. Gaberson & M. H. Oermann (Eds.), *Clinical teaching strategies in nursing* (3rd ed.) (pp. 151-181). New York, NY: Springer Publishing Company.

Chickering, A., & Gamson, Z. (1987, March). Seven principles of good practice in undergraduate education. *AAHE Bulletin, 39*(7), pp. 5-10.

Cioffi, J. (2001). Clinical simulations: Development and validation. *Nurse Education Today, 21*, 477-486.

Cordeau, M. A. (2010). The lived experience of clinical simulation of novice nursing students. *International Journal for Human Caring, 14*(2), 9-15.

Cunningham, D. (1996). Time after time. In W. Spinks (Ed.), Semiotics 95 (pp. 263-269). New York, NY: Lang Publishing.

Eggenberger, T., Keller, K., & Locsin, R. (2010). Value Caring Behaviors within Simulated Emergent Nursing Situations, *International Journal for Human Caring, 14*(2), 22-28.

Fountain, R. A., & Alfred, D. (2009). Student satisfaction with high-fidelity simulation: Does it correlate with learning styles? *Nursing Education Perspectives, 30*(2), 96-98.

Gaberson, K. B., & Oermann, M. H. (2010). Clinical teaching strategies in nursing (3rded.). New York, NY: Springer Publishing Company.

Gibbons, S., Adamo, G., Padden, D., Ricciardi, R., Graziano, M., Levine, E., & Hawkins, R. (2002). Clinical evaluation in advanced practice nursing education: Using standardized patients in health assessment. *Journal of Nursing Education, 41*(5), 215-221.

Goffman (1974). Frame Analysis: An Essay on the Organization of Experience. New York: Harper and Row.

Henneman, E. A., & Cunningham, H. (2005). Using clinical simulation to teach patient safety in an acute/critical nursing course. *Nurse Educator, 30*(4), 172-177.

Hotchkiss, M., Biddle, C., & Fallacaro, M. (2002). Assessing the authenticity of the human simulation experience in anesthesiology. *AANA Journal, 70*(6), 470-473.

International Nursing Association for Clinical Simulation and Learning, Board of Directors. (2011). Standard VI: The debriefing process. *Clinical Simulation in Nursing, 7*, S16-S17.

Ironside, P. M., & Jeffries, P. R. (2010) Using multiple-patient simulation experiences to foster clinical judgment. *Journal of Nursing Regulation, 1*(2), 38-41.

Jeffries, P. R. (2005, March/April). A framework for designing, implementing, and evaluating simulations used as teaching strategies in nursing. *Nursing Education Perspectives, 26*(2), 28-35.

Jeffries, P.R. (2007). Simulations in Nursing Education: From Conceptualization to Evaluation, the National League for Nursing, New York: New York.

Johnson, J., Zerwic, J., & Theis, S. (1999). Clinical simulation laboratory as an adjunct to clinical teaching. *Nurse Educator, 24*(5), 37-41.

Kirkpatrick, J., DeWitt-Weaver, D., & Yeager, L. (2005). Strategies for evaluating learning outcomes. In D. Billings & J. Halstead (Eds.), *Teaching in nursing: A guide for faculty* (pp367-384). Philadelphia, PA: W. B. Saunders.

Lauken, U. (1995). Modes of thinking: Reflection on psychological concepts. *Theory and Psychology, 5*(3), 401-428.

Leonard, B., Shuhaibar, E. L. H., & Chen, R. (2010). Nursing student perceptions of intraprofessional team education using high-fidelity simulation. *Journal of Nursing Education, 49*(11), 628-631.

McCurry, M. K., & Martins, D. C. (2010). Teaching undergraduate nursing research: A comparison of traditional and innovative approaches for success with millennial learners. *Journal of Nursing Education, 49*(5), 276-279.

Medley, C. F., & Horne, C. (2005). Using simulation technology for undergraduate nursing education. *Journal of Nursing Education, 44*(1), 31-34.

National League for Nursing. (2006).

National League for Nursing. (2012).

Parsh, B. (2010). Characteristics of effective simulated clinical experience instructors: Interviews with undergraduate nursing students. *Journal of Nursing Education, 49*(1), 569-572.

Rauen, C. (2001). Using simulation to teach critical thinking skills. *Critical Care Nursing Clinics of North America, 13*(1), 93-103.

Rauen, C. A. (2004). Simulation as a teaching strategy for nursing education and orientation in cardiac surgery. *Critical Care Nurse, 24*, 46-51.

Reese, C., Jeffries, P. R., & Engum, S. (2010). Learning Together: Using Simulations to Develop Nursing and Medical Student Collaboration, *Nursing Education Perspectives, 30*(2), 97-100.

Reese, C. E. (2010). *Effective teaching in clinical simulation: Development of the student perception of effective teaching in clinical simulation scale* (Unpublished doctoral dissertation). Indiana University School of Nursing, Indianapolis, IN.

Reilly, D. E., & Oermann, M.. (1990). *Behavioral objectives: Evaluation in nursing* (3rd ed.). New York, NY: National League for Nursing.

Seropian, M. (2003). General concepts in full scale simulation: Getting started. *Anesthesiology Analog, 97*, 1695-1705.

Shinnick, M. A., Woo, M., Horwich, T. B., & Steadman, R. (2011). Debriefing: The most important component in simulation? *Clinical Simulation in Nursing, 7*, e105-e111.

Swenty, C. F., & Eggleston, B. M. (2011). The evaluation of simulation in a baccalaureate nursing program. *Clinical Simulation in Nursing, 7*, e181-e187.

Vandrey, C., & Whitman, M. (2001). Simulator training for novice critical care nurses. *American Journal of Nursing, 101*(9), 24GG-24LL.

CHAPTER 4

DESIGNING SIMULATION SCENARIOS TO PROMOTE LEARNING

Diane S. Aschenbrenner, MS, APRN, BC, RN
Lesley Braun Milgrom, MSN, RN
Julie Settles MSN, ACNP-BC, CEN

"Good teaching is one-fourth preparation
and three-fourths theater."

—Gail Goodwin

INTRODUCTION

It is important for educators to understand the factors that structure and guide the development of a realistic and educationally sound simulation scenario. The NLN/Jeffries Simulation Framework presented in the prior chapter will provide the foundation for creating a well-crafted simulation. This chapter incorporates findings from the literature and the authors' cumulative years of experience in designing, conducting, and evaluating simulations.

Designing an evidence-based scenario requires forethought and preparation to portray a realistic patient story (Dowie & Phillips, 2011). The development of simulated experiences has been characterized as time-intensive (Lamontagne, McColgan, Fugiel, Woshinsky, & Hanrahan, 2008; Mould, White, & Gallager, 2011) and scenario writing in particular as anxiety-producing (Dowie & Phillips). To ease the workload, faculty can consider prepackaged scenarios from manikin vendors or textbook publishers that are evidence-based and validated. However, there are limitations to the ability to share these simulations. The program may be restricted to a specific manikin and purchased scenarios may not adequately address curricular components or areas of practice that faculty identify as vital for their program (Jarzemsky, McCarthy, & Ellis, 2010; Schiavenato, 2009; Waxman, 2010). There is a continued need for the development of clinical simulations and collaborative networks for educators to exchange scenarios. The following strategies and template are designed to facilitate the creation of a scenario that meets simulation standards of practice.

WHAT SIMULATION SHOULD I WRITE?

Simulations should be strategically integrated throughout the curriculum with consideration for the level of the student, course content, and meeting program outcomes. Begin by identifying the audience for the simulation and their current level within your program. Consider the knowledge and skills expected of the students at this point in the curriculum to be successful with the complexity of the simulation you are designing. Novice nursing students can gain confidence in performing a head-to-toe assessment on a manikin with programmed physical changes that have been learned in the classroom (Bremner, Aduddell, Bennett, & VanGeest, 2006), whereas senior nursing students have an advanced skill set and increased clinical reasoning skills to assess and manage the higher complexity of a deteriorating patient (Cooper et al., 2010).

The simulation scenario should represent a real-life patient care situation that allows students to advance their understanding, confidence, and competence relative to managing the condition when it occurs in clinical practice (Clapper, 2010; Morton, 1996; Mould et al., 2011). A clear connection between course objectives and the simulation scenario is recommended by Bremner et al. (2006) for best practice. The following questions should be contemplated when establishing the theme for your simulation:

- What focus is suitable, respectively, for a novice, intermediate, or advanced student?

- Should the simulation be interprofesssional?

- What are essential elements of a curriculum that you want to ensure for all students in the clinical setting?

- What are clinical situations that all students should experience but are not guaranteed at every clinical site?

- Are there required areas of clinical practice that are limited or unavailable to students?

- Are there conditions not frequently encountered that should be simulated to maintain competence in care or performed first in a safe environment?

- How can learning from the classroom be applied to the clinical setting through simulation?

- Are there simulations already available on this topic?

Instructors can draw from prior clinical experiences and creatively replicate the event in a simulation scenario to promote student learning. The situation should mimic clinical reality. To ensure the integrity of the simulation, clinical expertise on the topic of the scenario is necessary for an accurate depiction of the event and the intervention responses (Waxman, 2010). Consider whether you are the best person to write the scenario or if an expert in the topic area should be consulted.

As you select the theme for your simulation, once again consider the level of the student. Waxman and Telles (2009) propose that a simulation be designed using Benner's model of moving from novice to expert. As students progress through the curriculum, the simulation scenario should become more complex and draw on the knowledge they have learned in previous course work and clinical experiences. For example, the focus of a communication scenario appropriate for a beginning nursing student can involve an interaction with the patient and family to help advance proficiency with this skill. Interprofessional communication can be integrated into a simulation suitable for the intermediate-level student in which the student can gain practice calling a physician about a problem while also ensuring receipt of adequate orders to correct the condition. A communication experience for an advanced nursing student can incorporate a difficult conversation such as interacting with patients who have been told they have a terminal illness.

Consideration should be given to writing scenarios to promote student knowledge, skills, and abilities in areas that research indicates students demonstrate difficulty.

For example, in various studies students have been shown to be ineffective relative to recognizing deterioration of a patient's physical status, appropriately calling for assistance from other members of the health care team, and anticipating medical orders that might be forthcoming (Cooper et al., 2010; Fero et al., 2010). This indicates that creation of scenarios in which the students must practice inductive and comparative clinical reasoning and communicating with physicians and others on the health care team would be valuable.

Consider available scenario resources as you are selecting a topic. Code, respiratory, and heart failure themes are frequently chosen for scenario development and are already available. Jarzemsky et al. (2010) suggest strategies for incorporating Quality and Safety Education for Nurses (QSEN) competencies (Cronenwett et al., 2007) into a scenario design. A simulation incorporating these competencies that also meets course outcomes may already be developed and found on the QSEN website for you to retrieve. Such a resource may also spark an idea for a simulation.

Select the setting that is appropriate for the participants and the chosen topic. Scenarios are often written for the acute care environment, but faculty should consider a broader variety of settings for simulations, such as the home, outpatient, rehabilitation, or nursing home setting. Unsworth, Tuffnell, and Platt (2011) assert that there is an underuse of simulation in primary care situations. Their study suggests the use of community-based simulations created to assess the deterioration of a patient and determine if the patient could be safely managed at home. Additionally, an unfolding case can incorporate the transfer of a patient from one setting to another as the condition evolves, which may encompass more than one simulation scenario.

Decide if the simulation will be used as a formative or summative evaluation. A formative evaluation provides feedback for a person to improve. A summative evaluation certifies the competence of a person relative to attaining the learning objectives (National League for Nursing, n.d.).

The most important component for designing a simulation is the identification of clear learning objectives that drive the scenario and debriefing (Waxman, 2010). The scenario should be written to address predetermined learning objectives. For example, Jarzemsky et al. (2010) describe how the knowledge, skills, and attitudes competencies of QSEN guide the development of learning objectives, which then cue the key events of the simulation. The outlined objectives should reflect the students' experience level and exposure to the content (Speralazza & Cangelosi, 2009). Clear objectives and a suitable problem are two significant design characteristics described by Smith and Roehrs (2009) that educators should pay close attention to when developing a high-fidelity simulation.

General objectives are broad-based or standard and can be provided to the students (Henneman, Cunningham, Roche, & Curnin, 2007) without disclosing the specific components expected during a particular simulation. Examples are objectives relevant to communication, safety, and assessments, depending on the theme of the scenario. General or primary objectives can include core competencies of a course or program (Waxman, 2010). Specific objectives represent more explicit components of the scenario and entail more detailed student behaviors and decision-making that should occur in the simulation, which are also processed during debriefing (Henneman et al.).

It is best to keep the simulation simple as you begin to write the objectives. Four to five general and specific objectives can guide a successful simulation. Carefully consider the skills incorporated in the simulation so students can succeed in the timeframe allotted for the simulation. Consider how long the simulation will run. The authors' experiences favor 15- to 20-minute simulations, which is a guideline offered by McCausland, Curran, and Cataldi (2004), with the debriefing at least as long as the simulation. However, Cooper et al. (2010) describe seven-minute simulations for clinical skills. A model case for simulation presented by Dreifuerst (2009) describes a 20-minute simulation with a 40-minute debriefing and a borderline case with a 20-minute period for debriefing.

WRITE IT AND THEY WILL COME

After you have determined that you need to create a simulation (or modify one that was purchased or shared) to meet the needs of your students and your curriculum and after you have considered the level of student knowledge and abilities and created the desired objectives, the next step is to actually write the story.

As stated previously, knowledge and clinical expertise are needed to create a scenario that is realistic. Use your knowledge to create a patient situation that will assist the student in meeting desired objectives. Approach writing a scenario as you would approach writing a story or play. Every story has a beginning, middle, and ending. In the case of a simulation scenario, you should consider the beginning as everything that occurs before the students enter the room to start the simulation. The middle of the story is what occurs when the students are in the simulated patient experience. The ending or conclusion begins while the students are still in the simulation room and extends till the end of the debriefing session.

UNDERSTANDING THE PARTS OF THE STORY

The story itself is dependent on your desired objectives and focus. Consider three potential scenarios written about heart failure. For example, consider a story about a patient admitted yesterday to a general medical-surgical unit with exacerbation of chronic heart failure and started on treatment with IV diuretics. What is not yet known to the student is that the drug therapy has not been completely effective in controlling the acute exacerbation. These facts comprise the beginning of the story. The plot would then be that the student, playing the role of the nurse, would assess the patient's physical status and administer an additional dose of ordered diuretics. This would be the middle of the story. The expected ending of the story would be an increase in the patient's urinary output and clearer lung sounds. The patient would continue to improve and would be discharged home.

Contrast this to the story of a patient who is post-myocardial infarction (MI) and in the coronary care unit of the hospital. The nurse has just received a shift report that the patient is recovering from the MI. The nurse is to enter and begin a routine assessment. All of this information is presented at the beginning of the story. When the nurse performs a routine assessment the following is discovered: new onset of adventitious breath sounds, a decreased urinary output, a decrease in blood pressure, and an increase in pulse rate. The expected action of the learner would be to utilize knowledge (e.g., that acute heart failure is possible after an MI), recognize the signs and symptoms of heart failure, provide appropriate immediate care (such as raising the head of the bed), contact a physician or nurse practitioner to report the changes, and perhaps administer newly ordered medications. All of these events comprise the middle of the story. The expected ending of the story would be that the patient has a positive physiologic response (e.g., clear breath sounds, normalization of vital signs, and an increase in urinary output). The patient recovers from his myocardial infarction without the development of significant complications.

Finally, consider a third story of a patient with chronic heart failure who is receiving a visit from the home health nurse. The patient has been in and out of the hospital several times in the last three months with acute exacerbations of heart failure. The goal of the visit would be an assessment to determine potential reasons the patient has been hospitalized so frequently. This is the story's beginning. The nurse arrives at the patient's home and assesses adherence with drug therapy using a "brown bag" inventory of medications and assesses dietary compliance using a 24-hour recall of the foods eaten. The nurse learns that the patient has inadvertently eaten foods with high sodium content. The nurse then provides appropriate teaching to the patient and family. This is the middle of the story. The ideal end of the story would be that the patient and family understand the teaching provided by the nurse and make appropriate dietary changes. As a result, the patient's heart failure stabilizes and he does not require hospitalization again for a year or more.

In each of these cases the patient had heart failure, but the story was completely different and the learner would meet very different objectives in each of these simulations.

The story that is created must allow for the learner to have a key role in creating the outcome of the story. In other words, it must be an interactive and student-centered experience (Clapper, 2010). All of the story may not occur during the simulation. The rest of the story is incorporated into the debriefing discussion to complete the learning experience and provide a frame of reference for the experience. For example, if using the story of the patient post-MI who is showing evidence of developing heart failure, the student may get as far in the simulation as realizing that the patient shows signs of heart failure but does not contact the physician. The debriefing should include a discussion of what information would be shared with the physician and what new orders might be expected based on these new findings.

CONSIDERATIONS FOR THE BEGINNING OF THE STORY

Because a simulation scenario is time limited, it is important to determine where in the story the learner will enter. Whatever has occurred up to the point in time the student enters the room and begins to care for the patient is the beginning of the story. Some of this information might be provided prior to the day of the simulation (e.g., a posting of the "medical record" for the patient), and some of it may be provided only immediately before the simulation (e.g., a shift report given to the learner).

An important part of the beginning of the story is creation of the characters. All of the characters in the story are introduced in the beginning. The characters in your story must be fleshed out and developed into real people. The story board should not just be about "a patient who is post-Myocardial Infarction (MI)," but rather about Donnel Maddox who is 56 years old, African American, and Baptist. He developed chest pain at work and then collapsed. It is now three days post-acute MI and he is in the coronary care unit. Furthermore, as the author of the story, you need to avoid creating characters who are stereotyped or reflect personal biases.

The characters need to be described in enough detail to become real to the learners. Information such as age, race, religion, marital status, and occupation help to make the character real. Characters should be different ages, races, sexes, and of different backgrounds. In writing scenarios you should strive to create some patients who represent the population at large and some who will represent those encountered frequently in the portrayed work setting or the geographic region of your school or hospital. For example, consider making the patient with an MI hard of hearing in one ear or visually impaired. Or the patient could be physically handicapped and wheelchair bound. Perhaps the patient could have a history of alcohol abuse. Although it is possible that you might design a specific scenario with the sole purpose of highlighting the care variations required by some of these patients (e.g., the main objective of a scenario could be that the student is to demonstrate effective communication with a hearing-impaired patient), many times these variations can be added to scenarios simply to provide normal variations among patients. Character variations also provide additional complexity to the story.

In addition to this basic information, more nuanced or detailed information assists students in exploring how various people will respond in a given situation. This information will be provided to whomever is playing a particular role in a scenario, such as the spouse of the patient. All characters should be able to answer the following questions: What is their background? Why are they here? What is their current emotional state? What are their expectations from this interaction? There should be enough information provided so that all role players will be able to respond appropriately and authentically as the nurses interact with them. This information, however, should not be so extensive that the role players feel they must read a script. Neither should it be so extensive that role players veer away from the key objectives that are to be covered in the simulation scenario to bring forth all of this other information. An example of a storyline that may divert from the main objectives is a patient or family member who speaks a foreign language. If communicating with a language barrier is a specific objective then this is acceptable. If it is not one of your four or five specific objectives, careful consideration should be given to this design feature since a language barrier may prevent the student from meeting the predetermined objectives. This balance must be considered and accounted for in the development of the story and the materials provided to the learners in various roles. Creating a variety of patients and other characters brings additional depth and complexity to the scenario.

Casting for the role of the patient is another decision that must be made when writing the beginning of the story. Based on how the story unfolds and the objectives of the scenario, you must decide who or what will become the simulated patient. For some simulations, you may wish to use a standardized patient. For other scenarios, you may wish to use a high- or medium-fidelity manikin as the simulated patient. For some simulations, you might consider combining a task training model (such as an IV arm) with a standardized patient. Standardized patients are helpful when the key objectives of the simulation require communication skills, including nonverbal communication. Human patient simulators are appropriate when the key objectives involve recognition and appropriate response to physical changes within the patient, such as increased heart rate or decreased pulse.

Decisions about who (or what) is most appropriate to portray the patient must not only consider the story, but also the realities of the institution. Is there a pool of actors available to use as standardized patients? Are there funds available to pay for their services? Does your institution have the desired human patient simulator? The goals and/or the story line may need to be adjusted if your institution cannot provide the desired "patient" for your scenario.

Costumes, props, and the physical setting also play a part in the background of the story. Clothing that is scenario-specific for the patient, the family members, and the nurses is crucial. If the scenario takes place in a home setting, the patient and family member should be in age-appropriate street clothes. This is different from a story in which the action takes place in an acute care patient room where the patient wears a hospital gown. Students playing the part of the nurses should be dressed as they would in the actual patient care setting (e.g., in uniform in a medical-surgical unit or in a lab coat for an outpatient experience). Props that help make the experience more authentic need to be in the simulation room. For example, pictures of family members, water pitcher and glass on a bedside table, wigs or make-up on the simulated patient, a drain from a wound that has "blood" in it, or a Foley catheter with dark concentrated "urine" in it all provide background information to the learner. Incorporating the sense of smell will also improve the story-telling and the fidelity of the scenario. For example, does the home setting smell of smoke? Does the patient's hospital room smell as if the patient has an infected wound? Are there odors related to body fluids or body wastes that are present in the scenario?

CONSIDERATIONS FOR THE MIDDLE OF THE STORY

Once you have finalized the main story line, developed characters for your scenario, and set the stage, you need to carefully consider the story line and how to move the plot along to reach the desired outcome within your time constraints.

To develop a scenario that "mimics clinical reality," there must be complexity to the situation and some uncertainty as to the "proper" action on the part of the learner (Cioffi, 2001) (e.g., are the breath sounds abnormal enough to be concerned that the post-MI patient is developing acute heart failure, or do they just indicate that the patient needs to cough and deep breathe to prevent atelectasis?). The amount of uncertainty in a scenario needs to match the abilities of the learner to work through the situation. As learners progress in their ability from novice to beginner to expert, the scenarios should become more complex, drawing on the knowledge they have learned in previous course work and clinical experience (Waxman & Telles, 2009). A student in her or his first semester of school should have less uncertainty presented in the scenario than a student in the final semester of school. New graduates working in a hospital should have less ambiguity in their scenarios than nurses with several years of clinical practice and expertise.

To maximize the reality of the simulation as well as to tap into various learning styles to engage the student learner, the scenario story should be written to include auditory, visual, and kinesthetic aspects of learning (Clapper, 2010; Dunn & Dunn, 1993). Auditory aspects could include vocalizations by the patient, comments from the family, or typical environmental sounds (e.g., overhead paging, monitors beeping, an ambulance siren, TV sound track, or radio music). Visual learning cues may include the props set up in the beginning of the scenario or a change in the scene during the simulation, for example, the EKG pattern on the monitor changes. Kinesthetic activities require the learner to physically perform an action. Simulation scenarios can easily include this type of learning when the student completes a physical assessment, takes vital signs, administers a medication, or performs other psychomotor interventions.

Another important aspect to consider about the middle of the story is the running time for your story. How much time can be devoted to the middle of the story? The running time will be based on the objectives that need to be accomplished in this middle section of the story. As you write the middle of the story, consider how long will it take for the learners to perform the anticipated interventions. Practical factors will influence the selected running time. These factors include how long the simulation room is available and how much time is available for students to experience the simulation. Once you have determined the running time of the middle of the story, you next create a timeline of the expected sequence of action. What do you expect to happen the first five minutes of the simulation? The next five minutes? What should the students playing role of the nurses be doing? How should the patient and family respond?

Learners can sometimes get "stuck" in a scenario and fail to advance to the main point of the story. Or learners may get derailed by some aspect of the simulation and lose focus on their primary objective. As the author of the story, and the clinical expert on the content, you must try to anticipate these types of situations and have a plan for keeping the learner focused and working towards the objective of the simulation. Cues to guide the student back to the main focus of the simulation or to accomplish key tasks should be incorporated into the middle of the scenario story. Consider the following example. In the scenario in which the patient has been readmitted to a general medical surgical unit, the main goal of the scenario is for the learner to recognize that the patient has fluid volume overload from heart failure and to administer an appropriate drug that is ordered. But what if the learner playing the role of the nurse doesn't assess the patient's lungs but instead begins teaching about prescribed medications? In this case the learner will never meet the goal of the simulation because he or she doesn't realize there is an issue with fluid volume overload. A cue needs to be given to students at this point in time to redirect their attention. As the author of the scenario, you need to anticipate potential problems and plan out potential cues that can help the learner to refocus. In this example, the simulated patient could tell the nurse he could not talk much because of shortness of breath. Or the family member could point out that the patient appeared to be having more trouble breathing and ask the nurse to do something to help. Or maybe this could be the time that another team member (student) enters the room to help assess the patient.

Technical problems can also prevent a student from progressing in a scenario. For example, the student may have difficulty taking a blood pressure on the patient, and then spends the entire simulation time trying to figure out how to get a blood pressure. Or maybe the alarm on the patient's IV pump is beeping but the student doesn't know how to shut it off. The attention of all of the students in the room may shift to the beeping pump and they fail to see that the patient's clinical status is deteriorating and requires attention. In this case perhaps the patient or family member might offer a comment such as, "Oh, that beeps all the time. The nurse on the last shift was always hitting the reset button to get it to stop beeping and start working again." Often these responses must be improvised during the simulation itself.

Students can sometimes consider an intervention in a simulation that is not possible due to the constraints of the simulation. If these potential conflicts can be anticipated, they can be addressed in a way that does not violate the fidelity of the simulation. For example, if the student suggests ambulation to a patient manikin, the "patient" needs a plausible and ready excuse as to why it is not possible to ambulate right now. The answer should match the focus of the story and not derail it. These "patients" might respond that they are in too much pain to ambulate, too short of breath to ambulate, or that they just came back from walking around the nursing unit.

Though many potential problems of the learner can be anticipated, it is not possible to anticipate every possible action that the learner may take. Seropian et al. (2004) describe high-fidelity simulation as "inherently unpredictable," pointing out that the "physiology [of the simulated patient] is often dynamic and must be responsive to the actions of the students and other people in the scenario (p. 168)." The faculty member running the simulation, in addition to the faculty member writing the scenario, must also be content experts and know what would happen next in real life and be able to quickly adjust the scenario to incorporate these unpredictable events.

For example, a student in the scenario makes an inappropriate decision, such as selecting to give a patient demonstrating opioid overdose more morphine. In this case, there is no choice but to have the patient respond in a physiologically correct manner. Sometimes these unexpected decisions of the participants will require additional cueing or a physiological response less severe than it might be in the real world so that the scenario can progress and the real outcome can be addressed in debriefing or the scenario can be ended early. To continue with the previous example, if the student does not know what to do to correct a drop in the respiratory rate, she may decide to call for the respiratory arrest code team, instead of giving the ordered and available Naloxone. Since you had no intention of this story leading to a code you have no emergency response equipment easily available. It would be wiser to end the scenario and then discuss the actions in debriefing rather than to try to have a code scenario without any emergency response equipment.

CONSIDERATIONS FOR THE ENDING OF THE STORY

The end of the story occurs after the learner has interacted with the patient and family. It allows the learners to process the consequences of their actions. What is the short-term effect on the patient and family? What would be the long-term effects on the patient and family? Some of the ending to the story may occur in the simulation room, whereas other aspects may become evident during the debriefing period. The objectives written to guide the scenario action also help to guide the debriefing session. During debriefing students will reflect on their actions during the simulation.

Many times, however, a student never progresses far enough along in the story to reach the desired ending, but the allowed time period for the simulation has expired. In other words, the story is interrupted in the middle. To help students learn from the entire story, the potential ending or expected ending must be explored in the debriefing. In this situation, debriefing not only is a reflection on what did occur, but is also an opportunity for consideration of what would logically occur next in the story. Debriefing questions to guide this aspect of learning include: What would the nurse have done if there had been more time to continue? What would be the anticipated response of the patient to additional interventions?

Some particular objectives may be intended to be specifically met during the debriefing period. These include objectives concerning affective learning, such as exhibiting understanding or empathy for the family member whose loved one is seriously ill.

IS THE COMPLETED STORY EVIDENCE-BASED AND VALID?

The story should be written based upon up-to-date evidence such as from journal articles, clinical guidelines, and textbook information. The writer of the story should provide a list of references used as the evidence supporting the story development.

The story that is created must be checked for accuracy and fidelity. Is the basic premise of the story believable? Does it represent a patient experience that could actually occur? Are the expected interventions on the part of the nurse evidence-based? Are they realistic interventions for the nurse? Do they represent the current standard of care? Do they reflect the nurse's scope of practice? Are the physiologic changes in the patient realistic? Would a family member actually behave or think in the described manner?

The story should also be peer reviewed and/or reviewed by other content experts to confirm validity (Waxman, 2010). The story may need to be revised based on feedback from peer reviewers and other experts.

Cioffi (2001) cites the importance of content validity in the development of simulation scenarios. Content validity refers to the extent that a measure represents all dimensions of a topic. For example, does the story about a patient with acute exacerbation of heart failure capture all of the elements that would be present in a patient with this pathology? A variety of experts or judges should independently review and determine if all of the essential elements are present. High agreement among the judges lends credence to content validity. Face validity, which may be more commonly used in examining scenarios that are used at a single institution, does not require the more rigorous statistical approach that is required with content validity.

Piloting the Story

Once the story is written in full with a beginning, middle, and end, there is one additional phase to the creation of the story. The scenario needs to be piloted with a small group of learners who are the targeted population (such as second-semester nursing students or new graduate nurses). This is critical. How the students actually respond and think during the story can only be truly evaluated by having the targeted population experience the simulation scenario. The feedback from these students will help you to revise the story to be more effective. Piloting of the simulation scenario cannot occur with a group other than the desired targeted learners. It is not effective to have other faculty members or experienced nurses play the role of the beginning learners. Their perspective will be very different, and they will not be confused or misled by the same aspects that might affect a learner.

All information that is considered the beginning of the story needs to be provided to the learners in the pilot. This includes the objectives for the experience, any skills or knowledge that they are expected to already possess, the roles that they may be asked to play in the scenario, and whatever aspects of the beginning of the story that you want the learners to have (e.g., current medical record with orders, medication administration record, shift report information). Depending on the objectives and the story line, the information that makes up the beginning of the story may be provided to the learners some time in advance of the simulation (such as one or two days before) or immediately before the start of the simulation. Some authors refer to these activities as "pre-scenario" or "pre-simulation" activities for the learner (Waxman, 2010).

The pilot will provide valuable information to you regarding your story. You may learn from a pilot, for example, that it takes the learners much longer to move through the middle of the story than anticipated and you need to adjust the timeline. During the pilot you will observe first-hand if there are places in the story where the learner gets stuck or derailed. Additional cues can then be added to the scenario to prevent this from occurring. You may learn that there was a particular aspect of the story that confused the students. For example, if the patient was supposed to have fluid volume overload with insufficient urinary output but the Foley catheter and the intake and output records indicated that the patient had created 200 cc of urine in the last hour, the student may mistakenly assume the patient could not possibly have fluid volume overload. Adjustment of the patient records and the props for the beginning of the story are easy corrections to prevent future confusion. Piloting the scenario also can make clear that the objectives are unclear or unsuitable for the level of learner or that more background information is needed for the learner to perform adequately. Learner feedback is important to help those writing the simulation or running the simulation adjust the scenario to better meet the learning needs of the group (Waxman, 2010).

OVERALL REFLECTION ON THE STORY

Student outcomes from a simulated learning experience rely heavily on the quality of the simulation scenario. It is crucial to provide appropriate attention to the development of the story for the simulation. Too often the literature describes the use of simulation in a learner population but neglects to describe the scenario or how it was developed. Clapper (2010) describes how previous learning experiences may alter the perception of a current learning experience. This has important ramifications for those developing scenarios. It is important to create a story and scenario that not only provide a learning experience but also foster enjoyment of learning from simulated patient experiences. A well-developed scenario will not only help students be open to learning via simulation for this experience but for every future time they are asked to participate in a simulation.

Waxman and Telles (2009) point out that it is not only the learner who moves along Benner's continuum from novice to expert but also the faculty who develop scenarios for simulation and integrate simulation into their teaching. These faculty, though content experts, are initially novices in the pedagogy necessary for effective creation and implementation of a simulation scenario. Mentoring is needed during the process of learning to write and run simulations with learners.

THE VALUE OF A TEMPLATE

Consideration of all of the elements that should be incorporated into a simulation scenario can easily be overwhelming to the writer. To assist a novice in scenario writing, the use of a template is helpful to guarantee that no key elements are overlooked. Integration of all key elements is important in developing a valid scenario (Waxman, 2010). A template provides consistency among various users at a particular institution. The template also outlines an accepted format when scenarios are shared between institutions. Figure 4.1 represents the use of a template for the writing of a simulation scenario.

Figure 4-1 Example of a Simulation Template Completed with a Scenario

Title of Scenario: Medication Confusion in the Home Setting
Scenario overview
Indication for admission: Hypertension
Patient name: Kurt Henderson
Level of complexity: [core/complex] Core
Target groups: Undergraduate Nursing in Community Health course

Estimated scenario time: 20 minutes
Estimated debriefing time: 40 minutes

Brief Summary

[Approximately 3-8 lines providing the instructor with information about the diagnosis and condition of the patient, the progression of the scenario and the expected learner events/ correct treatment options]

This case presents a 68-year-old male with a history of hypertension, diabetes type II, renal insufficiency, and hyperlipidemia. He was discharged from the hospital two days ago and has confused similar sounding drugs, Cozaar and Zocor. He is scheduled for a home health nurse visit today.

The students are expected to recognize the presenting symptoms from an extra dose of Cozaar, which was takencorrectly last night at dinner time and then mistakenlyat bedtime instead ofZocor. The students should communicate the findings to the primary care provider and determine if the patient can be managed safely at home. Medication education and preparation of a safe medication administration system should be provided. The organizational error reporting systemshould be identified.

Educational Rationale and Need [a short text describing the rationale and purpose of the scenario]

It is important to provide adequate medication education to patients and resources for home prior to discharge from the hospital.The Institute for Safe Medication Practice (ISMP) provides a list of confused drug names reported through the ISMP National Medication Errors Reporting Program, identifying medications that require special safeguards to ensure patient safety. Recognizing and learning from errors is one of the approaches for improving patient safety as by reported by the Institute of Medicine.Students' exposure to a medication error in a simulated environment assists in recognizing strategies to reduce the risk of medication errors, monitoring for potential side effects of medications, managing side effects when they occur, and communicating a medication error. This can provide value to one's role in preventing errors.

Figure 4-1 Example of a Simulation Template Completed with a Scenario - con't.

Learning Objectives
General

X	[check relevant general learning objectives]
X	Identifies the primary nursing problem
	Identifies relevant patient history information
X	Implements patient safety measures
X	Explains physical findings and diagnostics related to patient condition
	Implements clinician orders appropriately
X	Implements interventions based on patient care needs
	Prioritizes nursing interventions
X	Identifies indications, contraindications, and potential adverse effects of prescribed medications
	Demonstrates correct medication administration
X	Provides relevant patient/family education and teaching
	Demonstrates therapeutic and confidential communication
X	Demonstrates direct and accurate communication with interprofessional team members
	Demonstrates effective team work

Scenario-focused [Insert 3-5 objectives specific to the diagnosis and treatment]

- Demonstrate a thorough patient assessment to identify a medication error
- Determine if the patient can be managed at home or requires hospitalization
- Communicate the error to the patient, family, and primary care provider
- Recognize factors that influence medication safety in the home and hospital setting
- Identify organizational error reporting systems that engage in root cause analysis and avoid blame

Nursing Diagnosis

Impaired peripheral perfusion related to an extra dose of antihypertensive medication causing hypotension

Lack of knowledge related to medication identification and side effects

Risk for falls related to fatigue and hypotension

Figure 4-1 Example of a Simulation Template Completed with a Scenario - con't.

NCLEX Test Plan Categories 2010	
Safe and Effective Care Environment	X
Management of Care	
Advance Directives	
Advocacy	
Case Management	
Client Rights	
Collaboration with Interdisciplinary Team	X
Concepts of Management	
Confidentiality/Information Security	
Consultation	
Continuity of Care	
Delegation	
Establishing Priorities	X
Ethical Practice	
Informed Consent	
Information Technology	
Legal Rights and Responsibilities	
Performance Improvement (Quality Improvement)	
Referrals	
Supervision	
Safety and Infection Control	
Accident/Injury Prevention	
Emergency Response Plan	
Ergonomic Principles	
Error Prevention	X
Handling Hazardous and Infectious Materials	
Home Safety	
Reporting of Incident/Event/Irregular Occurrence/Variance	X
Safe Use of Equipment	

Figure 4-1 Example of a Simulation Template Completed with a Scenario - con't.

Security Plan	
Standard Precautions/Transmission-Based Precautions/Surgical Asepsis	
Use of Restraint/Safety Devises	
Health Promotion and Maintenance	
Aging Process	
Ante/Intra/Postpartum and Newborn Care	
Developmental Stages and Transitions	
Health and Wellness	
Health Promotion/Disease Prevention	
Health Screening	
High Risk Behaviors	
Lifestyle Choices	
Principles of Teaching/Learning	
Self-Care	
Techniques of Physical Assessment	X
Psychosocial Integrity	
Abuse/Neglect	
Behavioral Interventions	
Chemical and Other Dependencies	
Coping Mechanisms	
Crisis Intervention	
Cultural Diversity	
End of Life Care	
Family Dynamics	
Grief and Loss	
Mental Health Concepts	
Religious and Spiritual Influences on Health	
Sensory/Perceptual Alterations	
Stress Management	
Support Systems	

Figure 4-1 Example of a Simulation Template Completed with a Scenario - con't.

Therapeutic Communications	X
Therapeutic Environment	
Physiological Integrity	
Basic Care and Comfort	
Assistive Devices	
Elimination	
Mobility/Immobility	
Non-Pharmacological Comfort Interventions	
Nutrition and Oral Hydration	
Personal Hygiene	
Rest and Sleep	
Pharmacological and Parenteral Therapies	
Adverse Effects/Contraindications/Side Effects/Interactions	X
Blood and Blood Products	
Central Venous Access Devices	
Dosage Calculation	
Expected Actions/Outcomes	
Medication Administration	
Parenteral/Intravenous Therapies	X
Pharmacological Pain Management	
Total Parenteral Nutrition	
Reduction of Risk Potential	
Changes/Abnormalities in Vital Signs	X
Diagnostic Tests	
Laboratory Values	
Potential for Alterations in Body Systems	
Potential for Complications of Diagnostic Tests/Treatments/Procedures	
Potential for Complications from Surgical Procedures and Health Alterations	
System Specific Assessment	
Therapeutic Procedures	
Physiological Adaptation	

Figure 4-1 Example of a Simulation Template Completed with a Scenario - con't.

Alterations in Body Systems	
Fluid and Electrolyte Imbalances	
Hemodynamics	X
Illness Management	
Medical Emergencies	
Pathophysiology	
Unexpected Response to Therapies	X

References / Additional Learner Materials

Cronenwett, L., Sherwood, G., Barnsteiner, J., Disch, J., Johnson, J., Mitchell, P., Sullivan, D. T., & Warren, J. (2007). Quality and safety education for nurses. *Nursing Outlook, 55*(3), 122-131.

Institute for Safe Medication Practice (2011) List of Confused Drug Names. Retrieved from www.ismp.org/tools/confuseddrugnames.pdf

Institute of Medicine (2003). *Health professions education: A bridge to quality.* Washington DC: National Academies Press.

National Research Council (2007). *Preventing Medication Errors: Quality Chasm Series.* Washington, DC: The National Academies Press.

Equipment Checklist
Medical supplies
- Empty pill dispenser for 7 days with two separate AM and two separate PM areas for pills.
- Blood pressure cuff at bedside table
- Thermometerat bedside table

Medications and Fluids
- Medication vial filled with 9 tablets labeled,
  - Cozaar (Losartan) 25 mg
  - TAKE ONE TABLET BY MOUTH TWO TIMES A DAY
- Medication vial filled with 6 tablets labeled,
  - Zocor (Simvastatin) 20 mg
  - TAKE ONE TABLET BY MOUTH ONCE A DAY AT BEDTIME
- Medication vial filled with 5 tablets labeled,
  - Hydrochlorothiazide 25 mg
  - TAKE ONE TABLET BY MOUTH ONE TIME A DAY

Figure 4-1 *Example of a Simulation Template Completed with a Scenario - con't.*

- Medication vial filled with 10 tablets labeled,
    - Metformin 500 mg PO BID
    - TAKE ONE TABLET BY MOUTH TWO TIMES A DAY WITH MORNING AND EVENING MEAL

Documentation Forms
- Notebook with blank form for report and assessment documentation
- List of medications with dose and frequency at beside table with the 4 vials

Preparation of Simulator and Environment
- Bedroom at home
- Patient dressed in pajamas in bed with head flat on pillow

Recommended Number and Role of Participants
Student roles
- Home health RN
- Home health RN on orientation
- Wife
- Two Observers

Instructor roles
- Physician by phone
- Pharmacist by phone

Description for student roles

Wife
You are the wife of Kurt Henderson and answer the door when the two nurses arrive. If they do not introduce themselves, you can ask, "Who are you?" You will tell them that your husband is still in bed and very tired. You are concerned about him. You have a blood pressure cuff, thermometer, four vials of medication, and a list of his four medications at the bedside table; if they ask for these. On a table in the bedroom, you have an empty medication dispenser that you just bought. After the nurses assess the patient, you can ask if they think he should be using a medication sorter. You should tell the nurse, "he has not taken his medications this morning. I was given a week's supply of medications when he was discharged two days ago, and there are five days of pills left. I plan on going to the pharmacy to fill his prescriptions tomorrow."

> ### Figure 4-1 Example of a Simulation Template Completed with a Scenario - con't.

Home health RN
You are a home health RN making the first visit to a patient who was discharged from the hospital two days ago with hypertension and diabetes type II. You are working with an RN who has many years of hospital experience but is new to your agency. You will be orienting this RN for one more week. Your home visit begins at 0800 after you receive report.

Home health RN on orientation
You are a home health RN on orientation, accompanied by a seasoned home health RN, providing the first visit to a patient who was discharged from the hospital two days ago with hypertension and diabetes type II. You have many years of hospital experience but are new to home health care and are on you last week of orientation Your home visit begins at 0800 after you receive report.

Observers
You are observing the participants and recording your evaluation of the simulation. Describe your observations and what you are considering as the simulation progresses. How thorough are the assessments and the communication? What would you do differently? You will provide your feedback during the debriefing.

Report to students

The time is 0800 and you are at Kurt Henderson's home about to knock on the door.

Kurt Henderson is a 68-year-old Caucasian male with a history of hypertension, diabetes type II, renal insufficiency, and hyperlipidemia. Four days ago he collapsed at home and was brought to the hospital. It was discovered that he had stopped taking his Lisinoprilafter developing an "annoying cough."A myocardial infarction and stroke were ruled out.He was discharged 2 days ago with a week's supply of Losartan (Cozaar) and Simvastatin (Zocor). These were added to the other medications he was already taking, hydrochlorothiazide (Hydrodiuril) and Metformin (Glucophage).Ahome visit by an RN was arranged for today.

Mr. Henderson's vital signs and labs upon hospital discharge two days ago were:
Temperature: 37° C; Pulse: 86; Respirations: 20; Blood Pressure: 124/78
Sodium: 137 mEq/L; Potassium:4.2mEq/L; Chloride: 99 mEq/L; BUN: 28 mg/dL;
Creatinine: 1.6 mEq/L; Glucose: 110 mg/dL;Hemoglobin A1C 6.5%

Medications are:
Cozaar (Losartan) 25 mg PO BID
Zocor (Simvastatin) 20 mg PO QHS
Hydrochlorothiazide 25 mg QD
Metformin 500 mg PO BID with meals

Figure 4-1 Example of a Simulation Template Completed with a Scenario - con't.

Simulator/Patient State at the beginning of the Scenario

Patient Vital Signs

- HR:124 regular
- RR:22
- BP:86/48
- Temp:37° C
- SpO2: 95%

Manikin Settings

- Auscultation sounds normal; pulses normal, lung sounds clear, bowel sounds normal.

Laboratory Data

Two days ago upon hospital discharge
Sodium: 137 mEq/L; Potassium: 4.2 mEq/L; Chloride: 99 mEq/L; BUN: 28 mg/dL;
Creatinine: 1.6 mEq/L; Glucose: 110 mg/dL; Hemoglobin A1C 6.5%

Patient Data

Gender: Male
Age: 68
Weight: 90kg
Height: 170 cm
Allergies: Penicillin

Past Medical History

Hypertension, Diabetes Type II, Renal Insufficiency, Hyperlipidemia diagnosed 3 years ago

Physicians Orders

[A list of orders, including information about whether they are available from the
beginning or should be provided during simulation. Use text from printouts.]

Scenario

Time	Monitor Settings	Patient/Monitor Actions	Student Interventions	Cue/Prompt
0 –7 minutes	Initial state: RR:22 HR: 124 regular BP: 86/48 SpO2: 95% Temp. 37°C Lungs clear Bowel sounds normal	"I am very tired. I am sorry I am still in bed." When asked, the patient is oriented to person, place and time. When RN asks about medications, "I did not take any pills this morning." If RN asks about meds taken yesterday, "Yesterday I took my usual water pill in the morning and diabetes pills with breakfast and dinner, And the new pills, I can't remember if it starts with C or Z, I took one in the morning, one with dinner, and one before I went to bed about 9 pm.	Introduce self . Identify patient. Wash hands. Begin Assessment. - Assess LOC and VS - Identify hypotension and tachycardia - Assess for orthostatic hypotension - Consider causes for symptoms - Review with patient and wife what medications have been taken, the dose, time. - Ask if a blood sugar was checked this morning. - Instruct the patient to hold the morning dose of Cozaar nddrochlorothiazide. - Check the medication listand vials to confirm the extra Zocortablet and one less Cozaar tablet; the patient took an extra dose of Cozaar last evening. - Explain the medication findings to the patient and family without blame. - Consider giving PO fluids	Wife:He usually gets up at 7 AM Why is he so tired? If RN asks about a blood sugar check, wife: " It was 108" After the RN checks vital signs, Wife:"Should I give him his morning pills?" After RN asks about medications, Wife: show the med list and point to the med vials If the nurse checks the number of pills in the vial, Wife: There should be enough pills for 5 days in those vials that we got from the hospital. I will be getting his prescriptions filled tomorrow.

Figure 4-1 Example of a Simulation Template Completed with a Scenario - con't.

Time	Monitor Settings	Patient/Monitor Actions	Student Interventions	Cue/Prompt
7-10 minutes	No change		- Call the primary care provider to report the findings using SBAR. - Determine if the patient can be managed at home or requires hospitalization. - Determine what medications should be held today and when to resume the Cozaar and HCTZ. Inform the patient and wife of the information received.	Physician: What are the vital signs? How does he look? Is he orthostatic? What is the blood sugar? Has he had anything to eat or drink? If no, have him eat and drink. Hold the Cozaar this AM and HCTZ for today; As long as the systolic BP is 110 or above, the PM dose of Cozaar can be given Do they have a BP cuff at home? Wife: Wife: What did the doctor say? It seemed like he was asking a lot of questions?

Figure 4-1 Example of a Simulation Template Completed with a Scenario - con't.

Time	Monitor Settings	Patient/Monitor Actions	Student Interventions	Cue/Prompt
10-20 minutes	HR 104 BP 94/50	Patient should ask what each medication does and repeat back a description of when to take the medications "I hope I don't keep confusing those medications."	- Formulate a plan of care to ensure patient safety. - Provide education on all four medications. - Plan medications around meal times and Zocor at bedtime. - Educate the patient and wife on med orders to withhold the HCTZ today and only take the Cozaar at dinner time if the systolic blood pressure (explained as the top number) is at least 110. - Explain that if the BP is ok, the Cozaar can be taken at dinner time. The Zocor is taken at bedtime. Take the Metformin as ordered. - Recheck the BP. - Assess the patient's/ wife's accuracy with taking a BP. - Provide both verbal and written instructions on medications. - Instruct on keeping a record of meds taken and call if a med is withheld. - Organize the pills in the medication dispenser having two PM areas, one for the pills with meals and one for the Zocor at bedtime. - Identify the organization's error reporting system to report the medication error.	When instructions are provided, Wife: Can you write that down? We are sometimes forgetful. I bought this medication dispenser, do you think I should put the pills in it or can you do this?

Figure 4-1 Example of a Simulation Template Completed with a Scenario - con't.

Proposed Correct Treatment

- Introduce self
- Identify patient
- Wash hands
- Assess level of consciousness and vital signs
  - Identify hypotension and tachycardia, but alert and oriented
  - Assess for orthostatic hypotension
- Consider etiology of symptoms
  - Review with patient and wife what medications have been taken, the dose, time
  - Ask if a blood sugar was checked this morning
  - Check the medication vials
- Identify medication error and communicate this to the patient and wife without blame
- Hold the morning antihypertensive meds
- Call the primary care provider to report the findings using SBAR
  - Determine that the patient can be managed at home
  - Clarify when to resume the Cozaar and Hydrochlorothiazide
- Give PO fluids
- Recheck BP
- Formulate a plan of care to ensure patient safety
  - Provide education on all 4 medications
  - Plan medications around meal times and bedtime
  - Provide verbal and written instructions on BP assessment prior to taking medications and when to hold the antihypertensive meds.
  - Assess the patient's or wife's ability to accurately take a BP
  - Instruct the patient and wife to keep a record of medications and call if they withhold a medication due to low BP
  - Organize the pills in the medication dispenser
- Identify the organization's error reporting system and Report the medication error

Figure 4-1 *Example of a Simulation Template Completed with a Scenario - con't.*

Case Considerations

[Based on the scenario-specific objectives, the case considerations should contain a short explanation about the proposed correct treatment]

The symptoms of tiredness and hypotension with a compensatory tachycardia should be recognized by a comprehensive patient assessment. The extra dose of Cozaar,an angiotensin II receptor antagonist that lowers blood pressure,should be identified as the cause of the symptoms. Other potential causes, such as low blood glucose should be evaluated. The patient can be managed at home after ensuring that he is stable and after aplan of care for blood pressure monitoring and withholding medication for hypotension is instituted. The nurse should also check that the patient is safe when out of bed and ambulating.

The medication error should be appropriately communicated to the primary care provider, patient, and family without placing blame. Preventive measures should be instituted to avoid a reoccurrence of the medication confusion. Patient and family education with written references to reinforce instructions on medications, the plan of care, and blood pressure monitoring should be provided.

The patient should be instructed to communicate with the health care provider if a medication is withheld due to a low blood pressure reading so the situation can be assessed and corrected.

Factors that influence medication safety in the home and hospital are: comprehensive discharge teaching with written reference instructions; prescription drug labeling guidelines; safety devices such as scanners, IV pump guardrails, and medication dispensing systems; computerized methods for identifying medications that require special safeguards, incorrect dosing, adverse drug interactions, allergies, and side effects; familiarity with the list of confused drug names reported through the ISMP National Medication Errors Reporting Program; and organizational error reporting systems that engage in root cause analysis and avoid blame. A pill dispenser, planning medications around meal times and bedtime, and keeping a record of medications taken or withheld are specific measures that can assist in medication safety for this patient.

Figure 4-1 Example of a Simulation Template Completed with a Scenario - con't.

Debriefing

Guided Reflection Questions

General Opening Questions	
	How did you feel during the care of a patient in the home setting?
	What do you think went well?
	If you were able to do this again, how would you handle the situation differently?
Scenario-Specific Questions	
	[case specific questions that do not fit under a QSEN categories]
	What were the potential causes for the symptoms the patient was experiencing? What did you identify as the actual cause? How does entering a patient's home to provide care differ from entering a patient's hospital room to provide care? How might it feel differently for a patient or family at home rather than in a hospital?
PCC	[questions related to patient centered care]
	How did you determine if the patient could safely be managed at home or required hospitalization?
T&C	[questions related to teamwork and communication]
	What did you communicate to the primary care provider? Describe your communication with the patient and family. Are there differences in communication strategies when you are in the community versus when you are in the hospital setting?
EBP	[questions related to evidence-based practice]
	What knowledge have you learned in your course work, your readings, or in clinical practice that helped you in this scenario?
QI	[questions related to quality improvement]
	How can root cause analysis of a medication error and avoidance of blame improve patient safety?
S	[questions related to safety]
	What are methods, devices, or standards of practice that influence medication safety in the home and hospital setting? What measures did you take to ensure medication safety for this patient? Are there other safety issues you consider when you enter a person's home to provide care?
I	[questions related to informatics]
	How are medication errors reported? How can information management systems assist with the quality and safety of patient care?
General Wrap-Up Questions	
	What have you learned from this simulation?
	How can you apply this learning to your future practice?
	Is there anything else you would like to discuss?

This template was adapted by S. Barry Issenberg, MD, FACP based on the Template for Simulation Patient Design, developed by Jeffrey M. Taekman, M.D. of Duke University and the Human Patient Simulation Template from the AAMC MedEdPortal. Used with Permission.

Summary

Although designing a simulation may initially seem intimidating to instructors, the process needs to be viewed simply as telling a realistic patient story. The simulation needs to have a clear starting point, enough tasks and decision-making to keep the simulation interesting, enough cues and fidelity to keep the simulation moving and realistic, and a predetermined desired end to the story. Using a template will ensure that these elements are in place. Expert review will provide face validity and the use of evidence-based content will create scenarios that are beneficial to all levels of students. Finally, a pilot test with the targeted group is an essential final element before using the scenario with real learners. Although there are several steps in creating a well-designed simulation, the outcome will benefit the learners as well as significantly reduce the stress on instructors during the simulation day. The positive outcome for both learners and instructors will ensure that both groups keep coming back for more.

REFERENCES

Bremner, M. N., Aduddell, K., Bennett, D. N., & VanGeest, J. B. (2006). The use of human patient simulators: Best practices with novice nursing students. *Nurse Educator, 31*(4), 170-174.

Cioffi, J. (2001). Clinical simulations: Development and validation. *Nurse Education Today, 21*, 477-486.

Clapper, T. C. (2010). Beyond Knowles: What those conducting simulation need to know about adult learning theory. *Clinical Simulation in Nursing, 6*, e7-e14.

Cooper, S., Kinsman, L., Buykx, P., McConnell-Henry, T., Endacott, R., & Scholes, J. (2010). Managing the deteriorating patient in a simulated environment: Nursing students' knowledge, skill and situation awareness. *Journal of Clinical Nursing, 19*, 2309-2318.

Cronenwett, L., Sherwood, G., Barnsteiner, J., Disch, J., Johnson, J., Mitchell, P., . . . Warren, J. (2007). Quality and safety education for nurses. *Nursing Outlook, 55*(3), 122-131.

Dowie, I., & Phillips, C. (2011). Supporting the lecturer to deliver high-fidelity simulation. *Nursing Standard, 25*(49), 35-40.

Dreifuerst, K. T. (2009). The essentials of debriefing in simulation learning: A concept analysis. *Nursing Education Perspectives, 30*(2), 109-114.

Dunn, R., & Dunn, K. (1993). *Teaching secondary students through their individual learning styles.* Boston, MA: Allyn & Bacon.

Fero, L. J., O'Donnell, J. M., Zullo, T. G., Dabbs, A. D., Kitutu, J., Samosky, J. T., & Hoffman, L. A. (2010). Critical thinking skills in nursing students: Comparison of simulation-based performance with metrics. *Journal of Advanced Nursing, 66*(10), 2182-2193.

Henneman, E. A., Cunningham, H., Roche, J. P., & Curnin, M. E. (2007). Human patient simulation: Teaching students to provide safe care. *Nurse Educator, 32*(5), 212-217.

Jarzemsky, P., McCarthy, J., & Ellis, N. (2010). Incorporating quality and safety education for nurses competencies in simulation scenario design. *Nurse Educator, 35*(2), 90-92.

Lamontagne, C., McColgan, J., Fugiel, L., Woshinsky, D., & Hanrahan, P. (2008). "What do we do now that we have SimMan® out of the box?" Using a template to develop simulation scenarios. *Clinical Simulation in Nursing, 4*(1), e35-e41.

McCausland, L. L., Curran, C. C., & Cataldi, P. (2004). Use of a human simulator for undergraduate nurse education. *International Journal of Nursing Education Scholarship, 1*(1), 1-17.

Morton, P. G. (1996). Academic education: Creating a laboratory that simulates the critical care environment. *Critical Care Nursing, 16*(6), 76-81.

Mould, J., White, H., & Gallagher, R. (2011). Evaluation of a critical care simulation series for undergraduate nursing students. *Contemporary Nurse, 38*(1-2), 180-190.

National League for Nursing. (n.d.). SIRC Glossary. In *http://sirc.nln.org* . Retrieved July 5, 2012, from http://sirc.nln.org/mod/glossary/view.php?id=183

Schiavenato, M. (2009). Reevaluating simulation in nursing education: Beyond the human patient simulator. *Journal of Nursing Education, 48*(7), 388-394.

Seropian, M. A., Brown, K., Gavilanes, J. S., & Driggers, B. (2004). Simulation: Not just a manikin. *Journal of Nursing Education, 43*(4), 164- 169.

Smith, S. J., & Roehrs, C. J. (2009). High-fidelity simulation: Factors correlated with nursing student satisfaction and self-confidence. *Nursing Education Perspectives, 30*(2), 74-78.

Speralazza, E., & Cangelosi, P. R. (2009). The power of pretend: Using simulation to teach end-of-life care. *Nurse Educator, 34*(6), 276-280.

Unsworth, J., Tuffnell, C., & Platt, A. (2011). Safer care at home: Use of simulation training to improve standards. *British Journal of Community Nursing, 16*(7), 334-339.

Waxman, K. T. (2010). The development of evidence-based clinical simulation scenarios: Guidelines for nurse educators. *Journal of Nursing Education, 49*(1), 29-35.

Waxman, K. T., & Telles, C. L. (2009). The use of Benner's framework in high-fidelity simulation faculty development: The Bay Area Simulation Collaborative model. *Clinical Simulation in Nursing, 5*, e231-e235.

CHAPTER 5
CURRICULUM INTEGRATION OF CLINICAL SIMULATION

Patricia Ravert, PhD, RN, CNE, ANEF, FAAN

*"…no industry in which human lives depend on
the skilled performance of responsible operators
has waited for unequivocal proof of the benefits
of simulation before embracing it ….
Neither should anesthesiology."*

–David M. Gaba, M.D.

This chapter will provide an approach for successful implementation of clinical simulations throughout nursing curricula. The approach includes a seven-phase map for success, including integration team formation, analysis, plan for implementation, development of resources, implementation of plan, evaluation, and plan revision and implementation.

Educators and researchers report implementation of a single simulation experience in a variety of courses of different curricula. Examples include a simulation experience in courses such as clinical foundations (Kardong-Edgren, Starkweather, & Ward, 2008), pediatrics (Lambton, 2008), community health (Yeager & Gotwals, 2010), episodic health challenges across the life span (Sinclair & Ferguson, 2009), psychiatric nursing (Hermanns, Lilly, & Crawley, 2011), senior capstone (Childs & Sepples, 2006), and an advanced practice course (Beauchesne & Douglas, 2011). Integration of simulation experiences in most courses in the curricula of various programs has been reported (Curtin & Dupuis, 2008; Garrett, MacPhee, & Jackson, 2010; Howard, Englert, Kameg, & Perozzi, 2011; Irwin, 2011; Schlairet, 2011; Seropian, Brown, Gavilanes, & Driggers, 2004). The experiences of the educators and researchers provide exemplars for successful curriculum integration of clinical simulations across a curriculum.

INTEGRATION TEAM FORMATION

As a program moves toward increased use of clinical simulation experiences, an integration team should be formed to oversee the process. The team functions to provide guidance in decisions regarding simulation and develops a plan for simulation integration. The team's role may include determining the settings in which simulation may be utilized, clarifying technology and computer use, overseeing fiscal opportunities and restraints, managing equipment acquisition, and creating policies such as scheduling of personnel and space. Once a decision is made to continue simulation integration, initially the team may meet weekly. As the integration is underway, the team may meet monthly or each term.

Successful teams include the "innovators" and "early adopters" of technology and simulation (Rogers, 2003). Members of the integration team should include a simulation champion (a team member that is very passionate, experienced, and willing to lead the simulation directive), an, administrative or academic leader, faculty and support staff members, operational personnel, and technology support personnel. Each member brings a different perspective to the discussions and decisions. The simulation champion is usually an "innovator" and may be the laboratory or simulation program director or a faculty member with a passion for simulation who is given release time from other responsibilities (Howard et al., 2011). The simulation champion is an essential player for successful integration because this individual brings simulation knowledge and and information that are helpful in the decision-making process regarding the promotion and adopttion of simulations and integration of experiences through the nursing program (Rogers). The champion also assists in integration by verbalizing and demonstrating the advantages of simulation experiences to faculty and staff. The administrative or academic leader's role is to approve funding and allocation of resources, define faculty and staff expectations regarding simulation, approve faculty release time or assignment, and interpret the regulatory stance concerning simulation in the nursing education program. The faculty members represent specific courses or work groups and provide insight into the unique needs of specific courses. Staff members offer information on the day-to-day functioning and scheduling of the areas to be used for simulation experiences. Operational and technology personnel provide the specialized technical expertise necessary to run and maintain computer and simulation equipment.

The integration team tasks may include reviewing simulation literature, visiting simulation centers to gather ideas regarding simulation resources and successful undertakings, analyzing the curriculum, identifying concepts to be achieved through simulation experiences, deciding where in the curriculum simulation experiences would best augment the content, and selecting a simulation framework. The integration team may also determine the simulation delivery model, including identifying the location where simulation experiences will occur (didactic classroom or laboratory), assessing resources, constructing participants schedules, creating simulation policies on scheduling and use of resources, developing goals and timeline, and designing the simulation integration and evaluation plan.

The selection of a simulation framework will provide a common language to guide discussion and decisions (Childs & Sepples, 2006; Irwin, 2011; Jansen, Berry, Brenner, Johnson, & Larson, 2010). Use of the NLN/Jeffries Simulation Framework provides a common language, and instruments have been developed to evaluate the simulation experiences based on the framework (Jeffries, 2005; Jeffries, 2007). The three instruments that are available from the National League for Nursing include the Simulation Design Scale, Educational Practices Questionnaire, and the Student Satisfaction and Self-Confidence in Learning tool (Jeffries, 2007)

The integration team must determine the model the program will use to deliver the simulation experiences (Childs & Sepples, 2006; Irwin, 2011; Lambton, 2008; Tuoriniemi & Schott-Baer, 2008). Most programs choose or modify one of the following four models: (a) all faculty are responsible to develop and execute the simulation experiences, (b) a core group of faculty is responsible to develop and execute the simulation experiences for all students in their course, (c) a champion or coordinator with technical and simulation knowledge skills works with content experts to develop multiple simulation experiences for various levels of nursing program and executes most experiences, or (d) a champion/coordinator works with content experts to develop simulation experiences and a core group of faculty or instructors execute and facilitate the experiences. Over time it has become apparent that the first model, expecting all faculty to develop and execute experiences, is rarely successful. Many faculty are uncomfortable with the simulation equipment, as well as the strategies, and require development and support to be successful (Jansen et al., 2010; Jones & Hegge, 2007). The last model has been most successful in full program integration because the simulation champion has oversight with adequate support of others to facilitate and deliver simulation experiences to many students in various courses. The integration team should review possible models and develop one that is suitable to the program's unique needs.

Another critical decision is whether the simulation experiences will be used as a teaching strategy or a summative assessment strategy. Most nursing programs use simulation experiences as a teaching/learning tool and as a formative assessment. Formative assessment provides ongoing review and observation of students and allows the faculty an opportunity to correct and mentor students. Although simulation is often touted as a "safe" environment to practice nursing care, students often experience anxiety about performance. If the decision is to use the simulation experience as a summative assessment the environment will not be considered a "safe environment" and students will be hesitant to try to provide care they are unsure of because they are being graded (Schlairet, 2011). If the decision is made to use the simulation experiences as a teaching/learning strategy in some cases and as a summative assessment in other cases, it is imperative that students know which type of experience they will be engaging in each time.

The development of the overall plan for integration is integral for success and is the responsibility of the integration team (Brooks, Moriarty, & Welyczko, 2010; Burke, 2010; Garrett, MacPhee, & Jackson, 2010; Hodge, Martin, Tavemier, Perea-Ryan, & Alcala-Van Houten, 2008; Irwin, 2011; Jansen et al., 2010; Seropian et al., 2004; Sinclair & Ferguson, 2009). The overall plan is developed during and after analysis and includes development of resources, implementation of plan, evaluation, and plan revision and implementation.

ANALYSIS

During the analysis phase, the team members should oversee a curriculum review. The purpose of the curriculum is to facilitate student learning to obtain the specific body of knowledge, attitudes, and skills necessary to practice as a registered nurse (Jeffries, 2005). Refer to Table 5-1 — Integration Team Questions. During the review, gaps in the curriculum may be uncovered and should be addressed. Faculty should determine where and when simulation encounters would best help to bring the information, knowledge, and practice for the students (Sauter, Gillespie, & Knepp, 2012).

The team should conduct an analysis of faculty and staff resources. The survey may seek to determine interest and abilities regarding use of simulation equipment and facilitating simulation experiences. Surveys often include questions to determine how simulation experiences are currently used. Simulation experiences can be used as part of a laboratory, theory/didactic, or clinical course. Sinclair and Ferguson (2009) used simulation experiences in place of part of the lecture content in an episodic health challenges across the life span course. Many programs use simulation experiences as part of the clinical and others as an augment to the student learning.

Part of the analysis should include an inventory of simulation equipment, supplies, and supporting tools. Faculty in different schools of nursing frequently have simulation equipment stored and not in use because of lack of training and faculty development on the devices, equipment, and the simulators. The inventory should investigate all types of simulation equipment such as CDs and/or DVDs (for education and training in curriculum content as well as instructions for equipment use), videotape/recording capabilities, task trainers (venipuncture arms, injection pads, models, etc.), manikins (including all levels of fidelity), medical supplies, and moulage supplies.

The administrative team member will analyze the resource needs for the implementation. The financial resources available will have bearing on acquisition of simulation equipment and supplies, as well as additional faculty and staff to support simulation experiences. Financial support for faculty and staff development are essential to success (Jones & Hegge, 2007; McCausland, Curran, and Cataldi, 2004; Medley & Horne, 2005). Faculty expenses may include funds for reduced workload while the simulation experiences are being created and initially used. The chosen model of delivery will affect the expenditures for faculty and staff.

During analysis, policies for laboratory and equipment use will need to be reviewed. Often existing simulation centers will share their policies and give the team ideas to discuss. Policies often include method of scheduling simulation experiences including space and equipment, priority of scheduling, confidentiality, student dress during simulation experiences, and use of simulation areas and equipment on weekends and evenings.

PLAN FOR IMPLEMENTATION

There is danger in purchasing simulation equipment without a plan for use (Seropian et al., 2004). Many programs have purchased equipment and it sits unused due to lack of trained faculty and staff and a plan of how to integrate simulation experiences into the courses and curriculum. Successful implementation requires a plan that is unique to the needs of the program (Brooks et al., 2010; Childs & Sepples, 2006; Curtin & Dupuis, 2008; Hodge et al., 2008; Howard et al., 2011; Irwin, 2011; Jansen et al., 2010; Mauro, 2009; Tuoriniemi & Schott-Baer, 2008). A good plan can overcome many of the challenges reported, such as faculty and staff knowledge deficit regarding operation of equipment and facilitation of simulation experiences, inadequate time to develop and carry out experiences, cost for purchase and maintenance, ongoing faculty and staff training, laboratory scheduling (web-based, if possible), space, and the logistics of providing experiences to a large number of students.

The overall plan will include the timeline for implementation of simulation experiences through the curriculum. Many programs plan for a two- or three-year implementation. Mauro (2009) suggests starting small and beginning with one type of patient case such as congestive heart failure, leveling the objectives according to course and student expectations as suggested by the Standards of Best Practice: Simulation published by the International Nursing Association for Clinical Simulation and Learning (2011). The same case can then be utilized in a more advanced course with higher level objectives such as developing and implementing a teaching plan and use of community resources. Others suggest beginning with one course and implementing one full simulation experience, then moving to the next course. See Table 5–2 – Example Abbreviated Curriculum Map. The first course may be chosen because the faculty members are enthusiastic and willing to adopt early.

Some programs have successfully implemented one or two simulation experiences in each course in a short period of time, such as over a semester, term, or school year. An aggressive plan such as this always includes significant faculty and staff development to the kick-off for simulation experiences.

The plan may also include a decision to emphasize particular concepts throughout the curriculum, such as the quality and safety competencies of patient-centered care, teamwork and collaboration, evidence-based practice, quality improvement practices, safety, and informatics. Refer to Table 5–3 – Example Plan to Build Concepts through Curriculum. If planned, simulation experiences can offer opportunities for learning and practicing interprofessional communication and teamwork (Benner, Sutphen, Leonard, & Day, 2010). The plan should include leveling of expectations according to course. With an emphasis on safety, a beginning course may focus on patient identification and the appropriate use of checklists, whereas an advanced course may emphasize the analysis of a simulated error and determine the root cause. The simulation experience for each course should be unique according to course objectives and student level but within an agreed upon format.

Most plans include a decision to use a standardized planning form or template such as the one in Chapter 4: Designing Simulations for Nursing Education. Using a standardized form facilitates the development of simulation experiences so all involved are communicating in a similar manner. The form also ensures all components are included during the plan for new experiences.

Scheduling of students is an essential plan component. Each program must determine if simulation experiences will be held as part of a scheduled laboratory time, during a clinical shift, or as an experience at the beginning or end of a course. Many variations have been effective. Many report that three to five students is the most successful group size in the simulation area at one time (Brooks et al., 2010; Childs & Sepples, 2006; Curtin & Dupuis, 2008; Howard et al., 2011). It is recommended to split a larger group into two smaller groups. While one group is engaged in the hands-on care, the second group may observe or be involved in a self-directed activity. The groups then trade activities and engage in the other experience. The schedule should also include adequate time for orientation to the simulator (if needed), running the scenario, guided reflection, and debriefing.

DEVELOPMENT OF RESOURCES

The plan should include time to make physical alterations, if needed, to the area where simulation experiences will occur. Some institutions install headwalls, video capture equipment, one-way mirrors, and storage areas to house equipment and supplies. Curtin and Dupuis (2008) described an integration plan with a limited budget that succeeded by using existing equipment, purchasing refurbished equipment, and slightly modifying existing space to accommodate the simulation experiences.

Faculty and staff development is of utmost importance. Unprepared faculty and staff lead to feelings of discomfort or anxiety and reluctance to participate in simulation experiences, as well as underused equipment (Benner et al., 2010; Garrett et al., 2010; Irwin, 2011; Jansen et al., 2010; Jones & Hegge, 2007). The faculty and staff development plan will depend on what delivery model is selected. If the delivery model includes a champion/coordinator who is a simulation expert or will be an expert with training, then the faculty/staff training will be different than in a model when all faculty are expected to use the computer with the simulator and facilitate experiences for their students. Depending on the expectations and faculty and staff roles, the development plan should account for the various needs. All faculty and staff will benefit from an overall understanding of the use of simulation experiences as a teaching-learning strategy, but if they are not expected to run the computers associated with the manikins then this training would be not be needed. The simulation champion/coordinator will assist, support, and guide the faculty and staff in their development. The faculty and staff development plan may include various formats, including brown-bag in-services, video conferences, online discussions, and workshops with hands-on practice (Jansen et al.). The goal of the training is to provide knowledge and experiences to develop the skills and confidence to effectively use simulation as a valuable teaching strategy.

IMPLEMENTATION OF PLAN

The integration team oversees the implementation of the simulation experiences. The implementation may occur over a school year or in most cases may take longer. Faculty should develop a reasonable timeline to facilitate the development and implementation of experiences. During the implementation, further faculty and staff development may be necessary. Some may find it beneficial to shadow an experienced faculty or staff member initially to build confidence in their abilities. As the simulation experiences are integrated into the curriculum, there will be unexpected challenges and the champion/coordinator will handle the day-to-day issues. The challenges and successes should be documented for review by the integration team during the scheduled meetings. The team should also review the timeline and determine next steps for implementation.

EVALUATION

An evaluation plan is essential to determine the success and outcome of integrating simulation experiences into the curriculum. Schlairet (2011) noted that without a plan the pedagogical improvement will not be captured and the impact will not be identified.

An ongoing evaluation plan may include assessment of faculty and student satisfaction, individual simulation experiences, identified curriculum gaps, and program outcomes (Bourke & Ihrke, 2012; Sauter et al., 2012). The instruments from the NLN simulation project provide evaluation data regarding the simulation design, educational practices, and student perceptions of satisfaction and confidence. Surveying the faculty and staff will provide insights into additional perceptions and bring to light concerns with the implementation.

The evaluation plan should include a method to determine if identified curricular gaps have been met with the implementation of clinical simulation experiences throughout the curriculum. The program outcomes should be re-evaluated to determine the impact of the simulation experiences as a teaching-learning strategy (Sauter et al., 2012).

PLAN REVISION AND IMPLEMENTATION

As the clinical simulations are integrated into the curriculum, an ongoing review of the implementation plan should occur. Part of the routine integration team meetings should include a review of concerns and issues, and evaluation results. The implementation plan should be revised as necessary. At the end of the school year, a careful review and plan revision should be completed to ensure continued success for the next school year. The team should review personnel needs and determine if assignments are appropriate or if additional personnel are needed for success. Further faculty and staff development (particularly for new personnel) may be necessary and should be included in the revised plan.

CONCLUSION

Executing a well-planned integration of clinical simulations into the curriculum is exciting and rewarding. This chapter provided a seven-phase map for successful integration, including integration team formation, analysis, plan for implementation, development of resources, implementation of plan, evaluation, and plan revision and implementation. A well-planned implementation is a reason for celebration. Successes and the effects on students and outcomes for the courses and program should be shared during program and course meetings.

Table 5-1 Integration Team Questions

What are your program outcomes?
What are the learning outcomes/objectives for each of the courses in the curriculum?
Are the learning outcomes/objectives being met fully?
Are the national nursing education initiatives incorporated in your curriculum?
What are the gaps?
What learning outcomes/objectives are currently being met through simulation experiences?
What learning outcomes/objectives are best met through simulation encounters?
What equipment and supplies are needed to provide the level of fidelity of simulation experiences to meet the students' need to obtain the knowledge, judgment, and skills necessary for safe, competent practice?
Where in the curriculum will simulation experiences be beneficial for the students?
What faculty and staff resources are available for integrating clinical simulation experiences?
Are technical and support staff available to assist in the integration and implementation of simulation?

Table 5-2 Example Abbreviated Curriculum Map

Placement	Concepts	Student Learning Objectives	Simulation Scenario
1st year	Assessment	Students will: Introduce themselves and check patient identification Perform baseline assessment. Document assessment findings.	Medical-surgical patient with uncomplicated hip replacement surgery
2nd Year	Communication	Students will: Note abnormal findings. Implement nursing interventions. Communicate findings, inventions, and patient status to health care provider using SBAR communication.*	Post-partum patient with increased bleeding and declining vital signs
3rd	Health Care Teamwork	Students will: Note and document abnormal laboratory findings Communicate with other health care team members (such as physician, pharmacist, dietician, and social worker). Document and execute plan of care.	Patient with tumor lysis syndrome

* SBAR = Situation-Background-Assessment-Recommendation communication

Table 5-3 Example Plan to Build Concepts Through Curriculum			
Concept	Beginning Students	Junior Students	Senior Students
QSEN/Safety	Follows appropriate guidelines for patient identification	Appropriately utilizes safety-enhancing technologies (such as barcodes, electronic medical records, and medication pumps)	Implements national patient safety initiatives and professional regulations in patient care simulations and clinical settings
Clinical Judgment	Gathers all data and information and attempts to attend to all. Learns what information is most important.	Attempts to prioritize information. Usually focuses on the most important information to develop the plan of care.	Using all pertinent data, develops appropriate plan of care. Implements plan with revisions as appropriate according to data.
Communication	Introduces self to patient and family. Listens to shift report and makes appropriate notes.	Explains patient condition to health care team. Gives end-of-shift report to oncoming nurse.	Discusses patient condition with health care team and patient. Uses SBAR communication.*

* SBAR = Situation-Background-Assessment-Recommendation communication

REFERENCES

Beauchesne, M. A., & Douglas, B. (2011). Simulation: Enhancing pediatric, advanced, practice nursing education. *Newborn & Infant Nursing Reviews, 11*(1), 28-34.

Benner, P., Sutphen, M., Leonard, V., & Day, L. (2010). *Educating nurses: A call for radical transformation.* San Francisco, CA: Jossey-Bass.

Bourke, M. P., & Ihrke, B. A. (2012). The evaluation process: An overview. In D. M. Billings & J. A. Halstead (Eds.), *Teaching in nursing: A guide for faculty* (4th ed.) (pp. 422-440). St Louis, MO: Elsevier Saunders.

Brooks, N., Moriarty, A., & Welyczko, N. (2010). Implementing simulated practice learning for nursing students. *Nursing Standard, 24*(20), 41-45.

Burke, P. M. (2010). A simulation case study from an instructional design framework. *Teaching and Learning in Nursing, 5*, 73-77.

Childs, J. C., & Sepples, S. (2006). Clinical teaching by simulation: Lessons learned from a complex patient care scenario. *Nursing Education Perspectives, 27*(3), 154-158.

Curtin, M. M., & Dupuis, M. D. (2008). Development of human patient simulation programs: Achieving big results with a small budget. *Journal of Nursing Education, 47*(11), 522-523.

Garrett, B., MacPhee, M., & Jackson, C., (2010). High-fidelity patient simulation: Considerations for effective learning. *Nursing Education Perspectives, 31*(5), 309-13.

Hermanns, M., Lilly, M. L., & Crawley, B. (2011). Using clinical simulation to enhance psychiatric nursing training of baccalaureate students. *Clinical Simulation in Nursing, 7*(2), e41-46. doi:10.1016/j.ecns.2010.05.001

Hodge, M., Martin, C. T., Tavemier, D., Perea-Ryan, M., & Alcala-Van Houten, L. (2008). Integrating simulation across the curriculum. *Nurse Educator, 33*(5), 210-214.

Howard, V. M., Englert, N., Kameg, K., Perozzi, K. (2011). Integration of simulation across the undergraduate curriculum: Student and faculty perspectives. *Clinical Simulation in Nursing, 7*(1), e1-10. doi:10.1016/j.ecns, 2009.10.004

International Nursing Association for Clinical Simulation and Learning, Board of Directors (2011, August). Standard III: Participant objectives. *Clinical Simulation in Nursing, 7*(4S), s10-s11. doi:10.1016/j.ecns.2011.05.007

Irwin, R. E. (2011). The diffusion of human patient simulation into an associate degree in nursing curriculum. *Teaching and Learning in Nursing, 6*(11), 153-158.

Jansen, D. A., Berry, C., Brenner, G. H., Johnson, N., & Larson, G. (2010). A collaborative project to influence nursing faculty interest in simulation. *Clinical Simulation in Nursing, 6*(6), e223-229. doi:10.1016/j.ecns.2009.08.006

Jeffries, P. R. (2005). A framework for designing, implementing, and evaluating: Simulations used as teaching strategies in nursing. *Nursing Education Perspectives, 26*(2), 96-103.

Jeffries, P. R. (Ed.). (2007). *Simulation in nursing education: From conceptualization to evaluation.* New York, NY: National League for Nursing.

Jones, A. L., & Hegge, M. (2007). Faculty comfort levels with simulation. *Clinical Simulation in Nursing Education, 3*(1), e15-e19.

Kardong-Edgren, S. E., Starkweather, A. R., & Ward, L. D. (2008). The integration of simulation into a clinical foundations of nursing course: Student and faculty perspectives. *International Journal of Nursing Education Scholarship, 5*(1), pp. 1-16.

Lambton, J. (2008). Integrating simulation into a pediatric nursing curriculum: A 25 percent solution? *Simulation in Healthcare, 3*(1), 53-57. doi:10.1097/SIH.06013e31815e9964

Mauro, A. M. P. (2009). Jumping on the simulation bandwagon: Getting started. Teaching and Learning in Nursing, 4, 30-33McCausland, L. L., Curran, C. C., & Cataldi, P. (2004). Use of a human patient simulator for undergraduate nurse education. International *Journal of Nursing Education Scholarship, 1*(1), 1-17.

Medley, C. F., & Horne, C. (2005). Using simulation technology for undergraduate nursing education. *Journal of Nursing Education, 44*(1), 31-34.

Sauter, M. K., Gillespie, N. N., & Knepp, A. (2012). Educational program evaluation. In D. M. Billings & J. A. Halstead (Eds.), *Teaching in nursing: A guide for faculty* (4th ed.) (pp. 503-549). St Louis, MO: Elsevier Saunders.

Schlairet, M. C. (2011). Simulation in an undergraduate nursing curriculum: Implementation and impact evaluation. *Journal of Nursing Education, 50*(10), 561-568.

Seropian, M., Brown, K., Gavilanes, J., & Driggers, B. (2004). An approach to simulation program development. *Journal of Nursing Education, 43*(4), 170-174.

Sinclair, B., & Ferguson, K. (2009). Integrating simulated teaching/learning strategies in undergraduate nursing education. *International Journal of Nursing Education Scholarship, 6*(1), Article 1, pp. 1-11.

Tuoriniemi, P., & Schott-Baer, D. (2008). Implementing a high-fidelity simulation program in a community college setting. *Nursing Education Perspectives, 29*(2), 105-109.

Yeager, S. T., & Gotwals, B. (2010). Incorporating high-fidelity simulation technology into community health nursing education. *Clinical Simulation in Nursing, 6*, e53-59. doi:10.1016/j.ecns.2009.07.004

CHAPTER 6

INTEGRATING GUIDED REFLECTION INTO SIMULATED LEARNING EXPERIENCES

Sharon I. Decker, PhD, RN, ANEF, FAAN

Kristina Thomas Dreifuerst, PhD, RN, ACNS-BC, CNE

"Teachers learn from their students' discussions."

—Rashi

This chapter was originally published in 2007. Although the philosophical underpinnings of reflection remain, its relevance to learning and clinical judgment continues to evolve. Reflection has been identified as a critical aspect of the development of clinical reasoning (Tanner, 2006) and the transfer of learning (Overstreet, 2010).

Health professions programs continue to be challenged to use expanding technologies and support innovations throughout the educational process (Benner, Sutphen, Leonard, & Day, 2010; Institute of Medicine [IOM], 2011). The Carnegie Study (Benner et al.,) recommended that nursing faculty implement teaching-learning strategies that engage the learner, promote self-discovery, require the application of concepts, and foster the ability to "think like a nurse." Moreover, these researchers note that "thinking like a nurse requires clinical reasoning, as well as critical, creative, scientific, and formal criterial reasoning" (p. 85). Recommended educational innovations include reforms in the methods, approaches, and settings used to provide clinical education. This includes patient-free learning environments such as simulation centers to enhance the training of health professionals while minimizing harm to patients (Ziv, Small, & Wolpe, 2000).

Consistent with the recommendation to be more innovative in educational practices, the National League for Nursing (NLN) (2003, 2005, Ard & Valiga, 2009) challenged faculty to be creative and design new methods for clinical education to prepare graduates to thrive in the ever-changing health care environment. Furthermore, the NLN stressed that these innovations must be research based and conducted in environments that enhance student learning. Studies on debriefing demonstrate that integration of guided reflection into simulation and clinical learning experiences is an innovative way to facilitate deeper student learning (Dreifuerst, 2012; Overstreet, 2010).

This chapter will present an overview of the concept of reflection, discuss the faculty's role in facilitating reflection, and provide a summary of the empirical findings to support the integration of guided reflection into learning experiences. Finally, this chapter will build on these data and present several frameworks to assist faculty in integrating guided reflection into simulated learning activities.

PHILOSOPHICAL UNDERPINNINGS AND DEFINITIONS OF REFLECTION

Dewey (1933) viewed reflection as an active, rigorous, and emotional initiative that promoted learning by building new knowledge on past experiences. He noted that reflection is caused by "a state of doubt, hesitation, [or] perplexity" (p. 12), requiring the learner to be open-minded and willing to engage in the process. Dewey believed the learner needed to recognize the significance of an experience and stressed, "One can think reflectively only when one is willing to endure suspense and to undergo the trouble of searching" (p. 16).

Dewey (1933) further divided the process of reflection into the following five phases: problem identification, collection of additional pertinent data, interpretation, hypothesis and reasoning, and testing or taking action. Problem identification could occur either during or after an experience and required both time and intellectualization. Once the problem is identified, the learner collects additional supporting data and evaluates it for relevancy. During the third phase, interpretation, the individual seeks explanations and resources to broaden the understanding of the experience. A hypothesis is formulated as understanding and insight are achieved through a critical analysis of the experience. This analysis leads to the final phase of testing, where the learner recognizes meaning and applies the acquired knowledge to new experiences.

Schön (1983), influenced by Dewey, describes two types of reflection: reflection-in-action and reflection-on-action. Reflection-in-action is the self-monitoring that occurs while an individual is engaged in an experience. This phase of reflection is stimulated by a puzzling or "interesting phenomenon with which the individual is trying to deal" (p. 50). Furthermore, Schön describes reflection-in-action as central to the "art" of practice. Reflection-in-action is the artistry displayed by the practitioner as knowledge from past experiences is integrated into an unfamiliar situation. By considering new situations in the context of being "both similar to and different from the familiar one" (p. 138), the practitioner can make sense of uncertain situations and respond immediately. Schön (1987) stated the level of this response is influenced by the structure of the institution, the profession's body of knowledge, and the competence of the practitioners.

Reflection-on-action (cognitive postmortem) is the conscious review of an interaction once it is completed. The goal of reflection-on-action is to critique an event in an effort to discover new understandings with the intent of applying the new knowledge to future practice (Schön, 1983). Dreifuerst (2009) identified reflection-beyond-action as the relationship between reflection and anticipation since the use of the understandings derived from reflection-on-action are applied to future experiences through assimilation and accommodation. This critical relationship between anticipation and reflection is essential to analytical and inferential decision-making.

Tanner (2006) notes that the clinical knowledge gained through reflection-on-action after an experience promotes clinical judgment; whereas, Decker (2007) found that senior nursing students who demonstrate the ability to reflect-in-action integrate knowledge from prior situations into their thinking process while providing care during simulation through assimilation of experiential knowledge.

Reflection is also a component of the cycle of experiential learning developed by Kolb (1984). The cycle of experiential learning provides a learning theory that integrates concrete (real-life) experiences, reflective observation (reflection or internalization of the experience), abstract conceptualization (looking for patterns and meanings), and active experimentation or building of new understandings. Kolb believed learning relied on reflective observations as an individual progressed from being involved to thinking about the experience and assimilating it into abstract concepts for future actions.

To summarize, Dewey (1933), Schön (1983, 1987), Dreifuerst (2009) and Kolb (1984) pose that reflection is an active process of self-monitoring initiated by a state of doubt or puzzlement that occurs during or after an experience. As an essential component of experiential learning, reflection promotes insightfulness, which leads to the discovery of new knowledge with the intent of applying this knowledge to future situations. This view is also supported in the nursing literature by Kuiper and Pesut (2004), who suggest that reflective thinking is necessary for meta-cognitive skill acquisition and clinical reasoning or judgment. This perspective is further shared by Ruth-Sahd (2003), who proposed that reflection decreased the gap between theory and practice. According to Dismukes, Gaba, and Howard (2006), meta-cognitive skills include the retrospective ability to critically analyze one's own performance, including "not just what went well and what went wrong, but why it went that way" (p. 23). Meta-cognition, or reflecting on thinking, is a form of self-regulation that involves executive reasoning which has a critical role in successful learning (Kuiper & Pesut).

Learning is not, however, guaranteed by the mere passage of time nor with experience alone (Benner, Hooper-Kyriakidis, & Stannard, 1999; Boud, Keogh, & Walker, 1985). It requires the learner to be engaged and reflective to acquire knowledge attainment from experience (Jarvis, 1992; Kuiper & Pesut, 2004; Wong, Kember, Chung & Yan, 1995). In fact, active engagement in the process is an antecedent of reflection (Rogers, 2001). Tanner (2006) and Teekman (2000) caution that learning from reflection is not automatic; it demands active involvement in a clinical experience and guidance throughout the reflective process. Summarily, the purpose of reflection is to integrate the new understanding gained from the process of review, consideration, introspection, and mindfulness to foster better actions and decisions in the future (Rogers).

REFLECTION AND RELEVANCE TO NURSING

The Carnegie Foundation (Benner et al., 2010) extended a call for radical transformation of nursing education to prepare learners for the complexities of the health care environment. This transformation requires educators to implement teaching strategies that capture the process of using knowledge (thinking-in-action), the ability to reason and adjust care as a situation unfolds (clinical reasoning-in-transition), reflection-on-action, and reflection-beyond-action.

The importance of guided reflection is supported by Murphy (2004), whose research demonstrated the instructional methodologies of articulation (oral and written) and focused reflection to assist learners to apply theory to the clinical setting and promote reasoning skills. Cato, Lasater, and Peeples (2009) demonstrate that students were able to engage in self-reflection and think deeply about simulated experiences after self-assessment and personalized feedback was provided using the Clinical Judgment Rubric (Lasater, 2007). This supports research by Conway (1998), which demonstrated that patient care varies according to the reflective abilities of the nurse. In that study, nurses who demonstrated minimal reflective abilities provided illness-oriented patient care, whereas nurses with reflective skills implemented care based on the individualized needs of the client.

There is also a perceived transferability of reflective practice to clinical practice when the former is integrated into an academic curriculum. Specifically, changes in clinical practice were influenced by increased assertiveness and self-awareness achieved through the educational experience (Paget, 2001).

In summary, the development of reflection as an art requires creativity and conscious self-evaluation over a period of time. Once developed, reflection allows the clinician to deal with unique situations and affects the quality of patient care provided. Therefore, nurse educators hypothesize that if simulated learning experiences are based on the principles of experiential learning, and guided reflection is embedded into the simulated learning experience, then the experience should promote the insight needed for the development of clinical judgment that promotes quality patient care. This hypothesis needs to be studied further and systematically, but the assumptions are sound and should influence our teaching process.

CHARACTERISTICS OF A REFLECTIVE THINKER

Dewey (1933) stressed that an individual must have a willingness to participate in the reflective process. Westberg and Jason (2001) share this perspective and add the characteristic of being willing to learn. Other experts described "the skills" required to engage in the reflective process, including monitoring, analyzing, predicting, evaluating (Pesut & Herman, 1999), and the ability to take risks, be open, and have imagination (Westberg & Jason). The following three types of reflectors have been identified: non-reflectors, reflectors, and critical reflectors (Mezirow, 1981; Decker, 2007). Non-reflectors have difficulty engaging in experiential learning and demonstrate difficulty with reflection-in-action. Reflectors are able to correlate isolated past experiences to the learning situation whereas critical reflectors seamlessly assimilate experiential knowledge while providing care. Further, the amount of facilitation necessary can vary according to the individual's stage of reflection. Non-reflectors require extensive guidance during debriefing and demonstrate limited ability to engage in reflection-on-action. Reflectors, however, engage in reflection-on-action but demonstrate some limited self-analysis and need some guidance during debriefing. Finally, critical reflectors actively self-analyze and identify specific areas for self-enhancement, thus requiring little guidance from a facilitator during debriefing (Mezirow; Decker).

REFLECTIVE THINKING: INITIATING FACTORS, BARRIERS, AND OUTCOMES

Factors that initiate the reflective process include a perplexing event that causes feelings of doubt (Dewey, 1933) or puzzlement (Schön, 1983). On the other hand, obstacles to engagement in the reflective process include prior negative educational experiences and an organizational culture that does not value the process (Glaze, 2002; Paget, 2001; Platzer, Blake, & Ashford, 2000).

Both negative and positive consequences of the reflective process have been identified, including a heightened perception of self-awareness (Henderson & Johnson, 2002), empathy (Gustafsson & Fagerberg, 2004), enhanced professional development, and building new knowledge upon existing knowledge and experience (Boud, 2001; Dewey, 1933; Schön, 1983). Clinicians who experience positive outcomes from the reflective process may even provide better patient care (Benner et al., 2010; Pesut & Herman, 1999).

Self-regulation and meta-cognition or reflection-on-thinking are essential elements for bringing together the knowledge, skill acquisition, ethical comportment and clinical experience that provide the foundation for development of expert nursing practice (Benner, 1984; Benner et al., 2010). Further, reflective practitioners are not just interested in what worked well, they are also curious about what did not work well in an effort to modify future actions to improve patient care. Benner et al. (1999) stated that reflection sensitized the learner to "context-sensitive patient responses" and the "meaning of specific responses" (p. 58), which promotes the development of clinical judgment and thus enhances patient care. Tanner (2006) also includes reflection as a critical component of thinking like a nurse, which informs clinical judgment and reasoning.

Negative outcomes of engaging in the reflective process include feelings of personal distress, self-doubt, isolation, and insecurity (Boud, 2001; Haddock, 1997; Kotzabassaki et al., 1997). In fact, the reflective process may not automatically promote learning and the development of insight without cognitive engagement. This is due to the reflective process "becoming diffuse and disparate so that conclusions or outcomes may not emerge" (Boud & Walker, 1998, p.193), and without appropriate guidance the desired outcomes of the reflective process may not be achieved.

Johns (2004) stressed that reflection can produce negative thoughts; therefore, the guide or facilitator needs to support the learner throughout the process. The role of the guide is to help the learner "think about things differently" (p. 77); to "infuse the practitioner with courage to take action to resolve contradictions" (p. 79); and to "... listen to the practitioner's story, ... and support the practitioner to face up to anxiety rather than defend against it ... to see beyond themselves, to reveal possibilities for responding in new, more effective ways within similar situations ... to nurture commitment and responsibility, [and] to challenge and support practitioners to act on new insights" (p. 74). To foster this experience, the guide needs to accept the relevance of the process and create a safe environment in which the expression of feelings and group interactions are supported and remain confidential (Ruth-Sahd, 2003). Table 6-1 presents features of a safe environment for guided reflection and Table 6-2 summarizes the key responsibilities of the facilitator during guided reflection.

Table 6-1 Facilitator's Guide for Establishing a Safe Environment for Reflection
1. Plan the experience as a learning opportunity based on specific objectives.
2. Select a tool or develop guiding questions to facilitate open discussion. (Faculty should use these as a guide for stimulating discussion; be flexible and process according to the learners' needs.)
3. Secure a private, comfortable environment.
4. Arrange seating in a circular design. (If this is not possible, modify the seating so that the faculty becomes a participant in the process, not the "controller.")
5. Limit participants to those directly involved in the simulated learning experience.
6. Allow time for reflection.
7. Introduce the session; emphasize the objectives and the importance of confidentiality and trust.
8. Allow for and facilitate open discussion between and among the questions.
9. Allow for periods of silence; give the learners time to think thoughtfully. (Wait time should be at least 5 to 10 seconds.)

Table 6-2 Facilitator's Responsibilities During Guided Reflection
1. Be supportive
2. Establish and uphold ground rules related to confidentiality and trust
3. Create an environment based on trust
4. Encourage and engage group members in dialogue
5. Listen attentively
6. Help the learner deal with feelings of ambiguity
7. Monitor and facilitate group dynamics
8. Promote the recognition of patterns
9. Facilitate the development of insight
10. Facilitate the transfer of knowledge
11. Nurture commitment to action
12. Challenge the learner to initiate change
13. Support the learner to act on her/his insights

(Carkhuff, 1996; Johns, 2004; Westberg & Jason, 2001)

The skills required to engage in the reflective process can be learned. But sufficient time and appropriate learning experiences (real or simulated) are needed to promote this process (Westberg & Jason, 2001). Development of insight could be lost if the learner is not allowed time to explore and connect the new learning. Therefore, nurse educators are challenged to plan learning experiences that (a) initiate feelings of perplexity, (b) require the learner to build upon past knowledge and skills, (c) require active participation in a patient care situation, (d) demand the engagement of critical thinking, and (e) support reflection (Westberg & Jason). The learning environment for these experiences needs to support a culture of trust and facilitate reflection-in-action, reflection-on-action, clinical reasoning-in-transition, and reflection-beyond-action.

FUTURE RESEARCH

Additional research is needed to provide the evidence that demonstrates the relationship between reflective learning and improved patient care outcomes when guided reflection is integrated into a simulated or clinical learning experience. This research could explore how the use of guided reflection impacts students' development of clinical judgment and reasoning throughout the curriculum. Other research questions are outlined in Table 6-3. These studies could explore the effect of nurse educators' commitment to evidence-based reflective teaching methods, as well as the outcomes achieved when innovative pedagogies and technology are integrated into nursing education.

Table 6-3 Research Questions to be Addressed When Integrating Reflection Into Simulated Learning Experiences
1. What conditions promote reflection during a simulated learning experience?
2. What are the benefits and risks of integrating reflection into a simulated learning experience for both the learner and the educator?
3. Does the integration of guided reflection into a simulated learning experience affect learning outcomes?
4. Does the integration of guided reflection into a simulated learning experience promote the development of clinical judgment?
5. Is insight gained during reflection transferred to the patient care setting? If so, how does this affect patient care outcomes?
6. Do past learning experiences impact the outcome of an experience that integrates guided reflection?
7. How do the various strategies used to promote reflection affect the learner's development of reflective thinking?

SUMMARY

A sense of responsibility, the ability to recognize the consequences of actions, and connection of actions with outcomes are required for an individual to engage in reflection (Tanner, 2006). The ability to think critically (cognition) and reflect thoughtfully (meta-cognition) are both required for clinical reasoning and judgment. Debriefing is a process that facilitates the re-examination of a simulated or clinical encounter to foster clinical reasoning and judgment through reflective learning. It also provides an opportunity for learners to reflect on their actions in a safe and supportive environment, assisting the learner in becoming a reflective practitioner (Dreifuerst, 2009). Furthermore, the process of engaging in reflective debriefing promotes knowledge attainment (Shinnick, Woo, Horwich, & Steadman, 2011), clinical judgment (Lasater, 2007), and clinical reasoning (Dreifuerst, 2012) which are desired outcomes in nursing education. Nurse educators have been challenged to be innovators in the process of educational reform to promote student learning and acquisition of competence. The integration of guided reflection into simulation and other clinical experiences could provide faculty with a unique strategy to meet this challenge while providing quality education. However, further research is still needed to demonstrate best practices for facilitating this process to achieve the desired educational outcomes.

REFERENCES

Ard, N., & Valiga, T. M. (Eds.) (2009). *Clinical nursing education: Current reflections.* New York, NY: National League for Nursing.

Benner, P. (1984). *From novice to expert: Excellence and power in clinical nursing practice.* Menlo Park, CA: Addison-Wesley.

Benner, P., Hooper-Kyriakidis, P., & Stannard, D. (1999). *Clinical wisdom and interventions in critical care: A thinking-in-action approach.* Philadelphia: W. B. Saunders.

Benner, P., Sutphen, M., Leonard, V., & Day, L. (2010). *Educating nurses: Acall for radical transformation.* SanFrancisco: Jossey-Bass.

Boud, D. (2001). Using journal writing to enhance reflective practice. *New Directions for Adult and Continuing Education, 90,* 9-17.

Boud, D., Keogh, R., & Walker, D. (1985). Promoting reflection in learning: A model. In D. Boud, R. Keogh, & D. Walker (Eds.), *Reflection: Turning experience into learning* (pp. 18-40). London: Routledge.

Boud, D.J. & Walker, D. (1998) Promoting reflection in professional courses: The challenge of context. *Studies in Higher Education, 23*(2), 191-206.

Carkhuff, M. H. (1996). Reflective learning: Work groups as learning groups. *Journal of Continuing Education in Nursing, 27*(5), 209-214.

Dewey, J. (1933). *How we think: A restatement of the relation of reflective thinking to the educative process.* Lexington, KY: D. C. Heath.

Dismukes, R. K., Gaba, D. M., & Howard, S. K. (2006). So many roads: Facilitated debriefing in health care. *Simulation in Healthcare, 1*(1), 23-25.

Dreifuerst, K. T. (2009). The essential of debriefing in simulation learning: A concept analysis. *Nursing Education Perspectives, 30*(2), 109-114.

Glaze, J. (2002). Stages in coming to terms with reflection: Student advanced nurse practitioners' perceptions of their reflective journeys. *Journal of Advanced Nursing, 37*(3), 265-272.

Gustafsson, C., & Fagerberg, I. (2004). Reflection, the way to professional development? *Journal of Clinical Nursing, 13*(3), 271-280.

Haddock, J. (1997). Reflection in groups: Contextual and theoretical considerations within nursing education and practice. *Nursing Education Today, 17,* 381-385.

Henderson, P., & Johnson, M. H. (2002). An innovative approach to developing the reflective skills of medical students. *BMC Medical Education, 2*(4), 1-4.

Jarvis, P. (1992). Reflective practice and nursing. *Nurse Education Today, 12*, 174-181.

Kolb, D. A. (1984). *Experiential learning: Experience as the source of learning and development*. Englewood Cliffs, NJ: Prentice-Hall.

Kotzabassaki, S., Panou, M., Domou, F., Karabagli, A., Koursopoulou, B., & Ikonomou, U. (1997). Nursing students' and faculty's perceptions of the characteristics of "best" and "worst" clinical teachers: A replication study. *Journal of Advanced Nursing, 26*, 817-824.

Kuiper, R. A., & Pesut, D. J. (2004). Promoting cognitive and metacognitive reflective reasoning skills in nursing practice: Self-regulated learning theory. *Journal of Advanced Nursing, 45*(4), 381-391.

Lasater, K. (2007). High-fidelity simulation and the development of clinical judgment: Students' experiences. *Journal of Nursing Education, 46*(6), 269-276.

Mezirow, J. (1981). *Transformative dimensions of adult learning*. San Francisco, CA: Jossey-Bass.

Murphy, J. I. (2004). Using focused reflection and articulation to promote clinical reasoning: An evidence-based teaching strategy. *Nursing Education Perspectives, 25*(5), 226-231.

National League for Nursing. (2003). Position statement: Innovation in nursing education: A call to reform. In *www.nln.org*. Retrieved July 5, 2012, from www.nln.org/aboutnln/PositionStatements/innovation.htm

National League for Nursing. (2005). Position statement: Transforming nursing education. In [www.nln.org]. RetrievedJuly 5, 2012], from www.nln.org/aboutnln/PositionStatements/transforming052005.pdf

Paget, T. (2001). Reflective practice and clinical outcomes: Practitioners' views on how reflective practice has influenced their clinical practice. *Journal of Clinical Nursing, 10*(2), 204-214.

Pesut, D. J., & Herman, J. (1999). *Clinical reasoning: The art and science of critical and creative thinking*. Albany, NY: Delmar.

Platzer, H., Blake, D., & Ashford, D. (2000). Barriers to learning from reflection: A study of the use of group work with post-registration nurses. *Journal of Advanced Nursing, 31*(5), 1001-1008.

Ruth-Sahd, L. A. (2003). Reflective practice: A critical analysis of data-based studies and implications for nursing education. *Journal of Nursing Education, 42*(11), 488-497.

Schön, D. A. (1983). *The reflective practitioner: How professionals think in action.* New York, NY: Basic Books.

Schön, D. A. (1987). *Educating the reflective practitioner.* Hoboken, NJ: Jossey-Bass.

Shinnick, M. A., Woo, M., Horwich, T. B., & Steadman, R. (2011). Debriefing: The most important component in simulation? *Clinical Simulation in Nursing, 7,* e105-e111.

Tanner, C. A. (2006). Thinking like a nurse: A research-based model of clinical judgment in nursing. *Journal of Nursing Education, 45*(6), 204-211.

Teekman, B. (2000). Exploring reflective thinking in nursing practice. *Journal of Advanced Nursing, 31*(5), 1125-1135.

Westberg, J., & Jason, H. (2001). *Fostering reflection and providing feedback.* New York, NY: Springer Publishing.

Wong, F. K. Y., Kember, D., Chung, L. Y. F., & Yan, L. (1995). Assessing the level of student reflection from reflective journals. *Journal of Advanced Nursing, 22,* 48-57.

Ziv, A., Small, S. D., & Wolpe, P. R. (2000). Patient safety and simulation-based medical education. *Medical Teacher, 22*(5), 489-495.

CHAPTER 7

DEBRIEFING: AN ESSENTIAL COMPONENT FOR LEARNING IN SIMULATION PEDAGOGY

Kristina Thomas Dreifuerst, PhD, RN, ACNS-BC, CNE
Sharon I. Decker, PhD, RN, ANEF, FAAN

"Education is not the filling of a pail

but the lighting of a fire."

–William Butler Yeats

Debriefing is an important component of clinical learning in practice settings and simulation environments (Dreifuerst, 2009; Shinnick, Woo, Horwich, & Steadman, 2011). With limited clinical time, inconsistent exposure to different types of patients, and variable interactions with faculty, nursing students may have few opportunities to link classroom content to clinical practice. Debriefing can be an opportunity to engage learners in the process of bridging content, knowledge, and experience through the use of facilitated reflection.

As the use of simulation pedagogy increases, debriefing methods continue to be developed to augment the experiential learning that occurs in these simulated clinical experiences. The importance of debriefing as an opportunity for learners to reflect on and interpret their performance in all types of simulation has been well documented (Cantrell, 2008; Fanning, & Gaba, 2007). This chapter will present an overview of the concept of debriefing, including several methods. It will also present research findings relevant to the use of debriefing methods and evidence-based principles of debriefing to support best practices in simulation and other clinical experiences.

OVERVIEW OF DEBRIEFING

Debriefing follows a simulated clinical experience to allow the students and instructors to revisit the encounter reflectively and learn from what happened (Arafeh, Hansen, & Nichols, 2010; Decker, 2007; Dreifuerst, 2009; Fanning & Gaba, 2007). It is a time to understand, analyze, and synthesize the thoughts, feelings, and actions that occurred during the simulation (Rudolph et al., 2008). While the format and process of debriefing can vary considerably, it is common for teachers and students to review an experience they shared, to determine what went right, what went wrong, and what should be done differently during the next simulation experience (Decker; Dreifuerst; Fanning & Gaba). These are elements of debriefing that have been adopted from its use in the military where it was important to receive a report or accounting of the details of a mission while at the same time providing an opportunity to allow the participants to release and deal with emotions related to the experience (Adler, Castro, & McGurk, 2009; Dismukes, Gaba, & Howard, 2006; Fanning & Gaba). Simulation debriefing is also derived from concepts of debriefing crisis situations where it has been common to debrief emergency service personnel to mitigate stress reactions following exposure to work-related trauma (Regehr, 2001). Using both of these traditions within an educational and healthcare framework, debriefing has been used extensively for the following three purposes: to receive an accounting, to mitigate emotional response, and to correct decisions and actions that were incorrectly applied in the simulation experience.

Debriefing is essential with all types of simulation. This includes low-fidelity case studies, medium-fidelity task trainers, and high-fidelity simulation involving the use

DEBRIEFING: AN ESSENTIAL COMPONENT FOR LEARNING IN SIMULATION PEDAGOGY

of computer-enhanced manikins that realistically represent the physiologic response of a patient in credible clinical environments. It is also appropriately used with virtual simulations, gaming and Internet-based clinical experience platforms, and live actor simulations. Debriefing has been shown to be critical for facilitating learning in simulation, particularly in the areas of cognitive development and decision-making (Shinnick, Woo, & Mentes, 2011). Since simulation represents simulated clinical experiences, it might then be inferred that debriefing traditional clinical experiences using similar methods and strategies could be critical for facilitating learning in that environment also (Dreifuerst, 2010). While post-conference discussions to summarize and discuss clinical are common in nursing education, research to explore the impact of debriefing methods in the clinical setting have not yet been published.

Debriefing is a constructivist, reflective teaching strategy and an essential component of all types of simulation which solidifies learning (Cantrell, 2008). It can be an occasion where clinical instructors encourage students to actively build upon prior learning and test assumptions about patient care and subsequent responses with the other participants in the simulation experience (Dreifuerst, 2009). This traditional model of simulation debriefing often includes a discussion between the teacher/coach/debriefing facilitator and the student(s) based on the intended learning objectives. In this typical approach, there is a focus on critique of performance prompted by asking the participants to describe what was done correctly, what was done incorrectly, and what they would do differently the next time (Decker, 2007; Flannagan, 2008). By answering these questions, students use inductive and deductive thinking skills that are foundational to critical thinking, along with simple analysis and basic reflection. In this manner, debriefing is similar to formative feedback for students based on evaluation of their performance during the simulation. It is this feedback that is intended to change behavior or clinical practice (Decker; Rudolph et al., 2008).

Differences exist between debriefing and student assessment. Debriefing can, however, use elements of formative and summative feedback, including clarification of a good performance (objectives, behavioral criteria, and expected standards), development of self-assessment, provision of high-quality information to students about their learning, dialog between teachers and students around learning, and an opportunity to close the gap between current and desired performance (Rudolph et al., 2008). When simulation occurs within a learning environment, the emphasis of debriefing is on understanding what occurred and discussing alternative actions and decisions. On the other hand, in those cases when simulation represents a formal evaluation, then assessment, critique, and grading of the student performance become the critical aspects and debriefing becomes a review of assessment findings.

Facilitation of debriefing is an important concept. Depending on the situation, the facilitator can be a mentor, coach, teacher, or peer. The role of facilitator is typically to

FROM CONCEPTUALIZATION TO EVALUATION 107

guide the debriefing experience. The level of involvement by the facilitator in the debriefing process is dependent on many things, including the ability of the participants to engage in autonomous reflection, the skill level of the participants, and the outcome of the simulation. Novice participants generally require more debriefing facilitation. Likewise, when there has been a highly charged or emotional experience or a negative outcome, a debriefing facilitator can provide support and instruction to foster positive learning from the experience (Dreifuerst, 2009; Fanning & Gaba, 2007). Facilitators can use many communication strategies, including open-ended questioning, active listening skills, Socratic questioning, rewording, positive reinforcement, rephrasing, pausing or deliberate silence, and guiding or leading questions. Skill in debriefing can require training and practice for best outcomes (Fanning & Gaba). Continuing education opportunities to learn debriefing are available from a variety of venues and may present overall, evidence-based debriefing principles or specific debriefing methods.

Best Practices

Although feedback and debriefing are recognized as critical elements in simulation-based education (McGaghie, Issenberg, Petrusa, & Scalese 2010; Raemer et al., 2011), a review of the literature demonstrated a need for studies focusing on the principles of debriefing (Raemer et al.; Fanning & Gaba, 2007). For example, the characteristics of good debriefing are seldom discussed in depth (Raemer et al.). Because of limited research-based findings, best practices for debriefing are predominantly based on observations and even trial-and-error rather than outcome data. Recognizing debriefing is critical in simulation-based learning and that the skills of the facilitator are learned and improved upon with feedback and reflection, faculty must be provided assistance and mentoring in developing this teaching skill.

This section will summarize the recommended best practices related to the following questions: (a) Who should facilitate the debrief? (b) What is the facilitator's role in the debriefing process? (c) What is the recommended length of a debrief session? (d) When should debrief occur? (e) Where should debrief occur? and (f) How should audio/visual recordings be integrated into debrief?

Who Should Facilitate the Debriefing?

The facilitators' competency in debriefing and their ability to engage the learners is important. It has a direct effect on the learner's ability to transfer knowledge and develop critical thinking skills (Seaman & Fellenz, 1989). Additionally, learners perceive an increase in learning when faculty who have a positive demeanor facilitate the debriefing (Cantrell, 2008; Lasater, 2007).

Facilitator competency is related to clinical competency. The debriefer should have the clinical knowledge and skills to care for the patient who is the focus of the simulation or clinical experience. This is important for several reasons. First, the facilitator needs to recognize whether the behaviors, decisions, and clinical outcomes that the learners demonstrated were appropriate. The facilitator also needs to be able to correct misinformation and poor choices with knowledgeable alternatives and corrected choices. Finally, the facilitator must be able to answer student questions about the clinical situation, the patient assessment, findings, and outcomes (Dieckmann, Friis, Lippert, & Ostergaard, 2009; Flannagan, 2008; Rudolph et al., 2008).

Debriefing should be facilitated by educators who observe the simulated experience directly or through video feed (Lasater, 2007; Wotton, Davis, Button, & Kelton, 2010). Observing the experience provides the facilitator a foundation to structure the debriefing and guide the discussion to highlight critical elements of the experience. An exception to this practice might be if both formative and summative assessments are integrated into the simulation or clinical experiences. In those situations, Wickers (2010) recommends that clinical instructors who are scheduled to conduct summative assessments not participate as debriefing facilitators during the formative assessments to prevent inadvertent influence in the evaluation process.

What is the Faculty's Role During the Debriefing Process?

During debriefing, educators function as both facilitators and instructors, guiding the learner to self-discovery while acknowledging any identified deficiencies (Rudolph et al., 2008). Facilitators should know the objectives and expectations of the participants in the simulation. Facilitators also need to know how to provide constructive feedback, respect others, listen attentively, and be considerate of the verbal and nonverbal communication occurring with the learners (Fanning & Gaba, 2007; Wickers, 2010).

Research conducted by Dieckmann et al. (2009) identified a correlation between the role learners play in a scenario and their engagement during debriefing. Individuals who were more active in the scenario were also the most active in the debriefing. Therefore, it is imperative that facilitators involve all learners in the clinical experience and the debriefing. Conducting debriefing requires "high diagnostic" and facilitation skills "to involve 'silent participants' without pushing them too much" (Dieckmann et al., e292). The ability to guide debrief requires a delicate balance in which facilitators support group interaction while at the same time facilitating self-reflection and regulation in the learners. Table 7-1 provides a list of educators' responsibilities during debriefing.

Table 7-1 Facilitator Responsibilities for Debriefing

- Review rules of conduct with participants
  - No cellular phones

  - Use respectful communication (brief learners on how to provide constructive feedback) (Arafeh, Hansen, & Nichols, 2010)

- Establish an environment of trust
  - Consider learners' cultural background, skills, and knowledge level (Wickers, 2010)

- Acquire confidentiality agreements (confidentiality protects learners, as well as the proprietary information of the program and curricula) (Arafeh, Hansen, & Nichols)

- Review learning objectives

- Set expectations for the debriefing session

- Facilitate the session according to learners' level of engagement
  - Keep the discussion learner-centered

  - Use active listening skills to encourage participation — eye contact, smiling, nodding, and utilizing therapeutic communication skills such as "Tell me more"

  - Ask open-ended questions (use these question to assist learners in seeing patterns and extracting meaning; avoid answering your own questions)

- Engage interaction between all learners (specifically, focus specific questions to silent participants)

- Use audio/visual aids to provide positive reinforcement and encourage analysis

- Provide constructive feedback and integrate instructional points at the end of the session
  - Summarize and reinforce the learning at the end of the session (Jeffries, 2005; Van Heukelon, Begaz, & Treat, 2010).

- Things to Avoid
  - Lecturing, whichprevents the learner for self-analysis (Fanning & Gaba, 2007)

  - Interrogating, ridicule, or blame. These behaviors stop discussion and prevent the development of insight (Overstreet, 2010)

  - Using closed-ended questions. Closed-ended questions limit deep thinking (Fanning & Gaba)

WHAT IS THE RECOMMENDED LENGTH FOR DEBRIEFING?

The length of time spent debriefing depends on the type and objectives of the simulation or clinical experience. Simulations that are brief and related to simple clinical situations and skill demonstrations may only require constructive feedback throughout the activity. Whereas simulations for complex care situations or clinical scenarios that are emotionally charged require longer time for debriefing. The initial 2003-2006 NLN/Laerdal study recommended the use of 20-minute scenarios followed by a 20-minute debrief or debrief sessions lasting as long as or longer than the simulated experience (Jeffries & Rizzolo, 2006; Wotton et al., 2010). Others recommended a period of two to four times longer than the scenario to allow students time to think deeper and engage in critical reflective analysis of the behaviors, decisions, and patient outcomes (Arafeh et al., 2010; Dreifuerst, 2012; Waxman, 2010; Wotton et al.). Clearly, the objectives of the simulation, the level of learner or participant, the behaviors, decisions and outcomes of the clinical experience, and the time constraints inherent in the schedule all impact debriefing time. In general though, participants need time and guidance to focus their thinking, analyze actions, hypothesize how the situation could be enhanced, and develop plans to promote additional learning. More research into this area is warranted.

WHEN SHOULD DEBRIEF OCCUR?

Debriefing occurs most often after the simulation or clinical experience has ended and the participants have moved out of the clinical environment. Post-scenario debriefing allows participants to experience the activity completely in real time without interruptions and lets the learner experience the consequences of behaviors and decisions by experiencing the patient outcomes. Additionally, learners have a tendency to begin self-analysis immediately following a simulation. Post-scenario debrief provides an opportunity to capture this and build upon this analysis (Cantrell, 2008; Fanning & Gaba, 2007).

However, facilitators may elect to provide debriefing "in-scenario" or upon suspension of the simulated experience if critical errors are made, when behaviors need to be corrected immediately, or when exemplary teaching opportunities occur (Decker, Gore, & Feken, 2011; Fanning & Gaba, 2007; VanHeukelom, , Begaz, & Treat, 2010). If critical errors occur, the ability to suspend the scenario provides an opportunity to mitigate negative learning that could develop when learners are allowed to proceed with the experience.

WHERE SHOULD DEBRIEFING OCCUR?

The optimal environment for debriefing is comfortable, private, and promotes trust and inclusiveness (Waxman, 2010; Wickers, 2010). Participants should be encouraged to separate themselves from the clinical environment and get comfortable to engage in active learning. Seating for the participants varies with style and facilitation method. For example, faculty might sit among the participants when facilitating small groups or elect to be at "the head of the table" for larger groups. A debriefing room or area with a white board or smart board may also be desired (Dreifuerst, 2010). In those cases, the facilitator or a participant might be standing away from the others to use it as a visual aspect of debriefing.

There are, however, circumstances when debriefing occurs in the clinical or simulation setting. This is often when the debriefing must happen "in-scenario" to correct actions or decisions immediately (Decker et al., 2011; Fanning & Gaba, 2007; Van Heukelom et al.,

2010). When this situation arises, privacy is essential and the facilitator may need to take the initiative to ensure this. A consequence of debriefing in the clinical or simulation setting is that participants may remain engaged in the clinical scenario and care of the patient, and thus are not actively engaged in the reflective debriefing process and learning may be impacted.

HOW SHOULD AUDIO/VISUAL RECORDINGS BE INTEGRATED INTO DEBRIEFING?

One study comparing the use of video recording during debriefing demonstrated no significant differences in student learning or satisfaction whether they are used or not (Raemer et al., 2011). The literature on this subject is mixed, however, and there is not enough evidence to support a definitive conclusion onthe impact of recording on student outcomes. If a clinical experience or debriefing is to be recorded, participants should sign consent prior to the experience. Additionally, individuals need to be informed of the center's policies related to use of recordings beyond debriefing, such as in professional presentations or available archives for later viewing.

The use of video requires faculty and staff to become proficient with the equipment. Depending on what is used, segments to be shown during debriefing can be indexed during the scenario and shown during debriefing to stimulate discussion. Only two to four segments should be shown which can be key debriefing points or examples of both good behaviors and actions that need addressing (Wickers, 2010). Faculty should introduce the expectation or goal for each of the segments, show the segment, pause, and allow the learners to self-critique and discuss. Finally, video recording of the clinical experience and/or the debriefing provides faculty with an objective record of the learner's performance that can be used for evaluation or integrated into the student's electronic portfolio.

SUMMARY

Recognizing that the ultimate goal of debriefing is to promote reflective thinking and assist learners in transferring skills from the simulated environment to actual patient care, it is imperative that best practices be established. Further research is needed to provide evidence that will assist educators in determining the most appropriate debriefing techniques for different learning objectives, scenarios, and learners. It will also be important to determine the optimal timeframe and environment for conducting debriefing.

DEBRIEFING METHODS

There are many different debriefing methods and strategies that are used in health care simulations. While similar attributes are found in many, each has unique qualities that appeal to different situations and learners. Six examples of debriefing methods are included in this chapter. This is in no way an exhaustive list of the debriefing methods that are currently used, but instead provides examples of some that are commonly used in health care simulation.

ADVOCACY-INQUIRY

The Advocacy-Inquiry debriefing method is used in the Debriefing with Good Judgment method (Rudolph et al., 2007). In this method, the instructor identifies a component of the simulation to explore further, many times because the student involved in the experience has done something unexpected or unanticipated. The advocacy is framed as an assertion or observation that is coupled with the inquiry or question. In this manner, the instructor is seeking more information and clarity about what occurred from the student in a nonthreatening way. The instructor's thoughts and judgment are evident to the student within the advocacy portion of the question. However, by coupling it with an element of inquiry, the student's perspective and dialog about her or his thinking and actions are valued and learning is improved (Rudolph et al.).

PLUS DELTA (+/Δ)

Plus Delta is a popular debriefing method for aviation and interdisciplinary health care simulation. When this method of debriefing is used, the simulation participants and observers create two columns or headings and identify positive actions and decisions in the plus column and things that could be done better or differently in the delta column (delta is the Greek symbol meaning change) (Fanning & Gaba, 2007). This method is not difficult and can be accomplished very quickly by a single participant or many. Nurses and physicians have readily adopted this method because of its adaptability to a wide variety of simulations. A debriefing facilitator can be present or team members can use this method without a facilitator.

DEBRIEFING FOR MEANINGFUL LEARNING©

Debriefing for Meaningful Learning (DML) is a method that uses reflection-in-action, reflection-on-action, and reflection-beyond-action to teach clinical reasoning and thinking like a nurse (Dreifuerst, 2009; Schön, 1983; Tanner, 2006). A premise of this method is that debriefing is a form of clinical teaching; therefore, having a clinical teacher with knowledge about the patient population lead the debriefing is an important consideration. While many debriefing methods use an open or semi-structured discussion, DML uses a consistent structure each time with nursing students to present and reinforce the process of thinking like a nurse (Dreifuerst, 2012).

DML uses a worksheet that provides visual learning opportunities for students, as well as a written record of the experience which they can take with them for review or reference. DML uses six phases in the debriefing process which were adapted from the E-5 model developed by Bybee and colleagues in 1989. Those phases include Engaging, Exploring, Explaining, Elaborating, Evaluating and Extending, which are iterative and often overlap during the course of the debriefing (Dreifuerst, 2010). Throughout the debriefing, the clinical teacher uses Socratic questioning to reveal the student thinking and decision-making that was behind the actions that occurred during the simulation. A focus of this method is ensuring that there is congruency between the actions, decisions, and thinking by the students. DML is a debriefing method that was designed for use with pre-licensure students because it focuses on learning to think like a nurse and development of clinical reasoning skills. It could, however, be adapted slightly to be successful with graduate nurses and interprofessional health care students.

GATHER-ANALYZE-SUMMARIZE (GAS)

The Gather-Analyze-Summarize (GAS) method uses a three-step process to guide the debriefing process (American Heart Association, 2010). Participants are first encouraged to make all of the information about the simulation experience evident by recounting events, behaviors, decisions, and outcomes. These can be listed in written form or verbally discussed. Next the participants and facilitator analyze all of the information that has been gathered. Analysis can be focused on the simulation objectives, the outcomes, the positive and negative aspects of the experience, and the actions or behaviors that were demonstrated. The GAS debriefing ends with a summary to reinforce learning. A debriefing facilitator can be present or team members can use this method as peers without a facilitator.

GUIDED REFLECTION

Schön (1987) proposed the use of a reflective practicum to enhance the process of reflection. A reflective practicum is a realistic event strategically planned by faculty to promote professional artistry. The environment for this learning event is described as being similar to those created in studios. Schön feels this unique environment allows "freedom to learn by doing in a setting relatively low in risk, with access to coaches who initiate students into the 'traditions of the calling' and help them, by 'the right kind of telling,' to see on their own behalf and in their own way what they need most to see" (p. 17). This reflective practicum has considerable likeness to the learning environment and experience depicted by the simulation framework proposed by Jeffries (2005). The simulation framework discussed in Chapter 3 emphasizes that for learning to be successful, the experience needs to be designed around the characteristics of objectives, fidelity, problem solving, cueing, questioning, and debriefing.

STRATEGIES TO GUIDE REFLECTION

Guided reflection can be integrated into the simulated experience to promote reflection-in-action, reflection-on-action, clinical reasoning-in-transition, and reflection-beyond-action through the use of Socratic questioning. The principles of Socratic questioning allow for the complexity of questions to be elevated as students acquire knowledge and skills (Benner, Sutphen, Leonard, & Day, 2010; Caputi & Engelmann, 2007). Several questions need to be developed prior to the experience, based on the intended focus of the discussion. Faculty could write these on prompt cards and strategically integrate them into the session to stimulate reflective thought. These probing questions should be based on the learning objectives and the abilities of the students, and should guide the learners' thinking. Faculty need to remember thinking is driven by questioning, but the quality of the question and how it is posed will determine the breadth and depth of the learners' thinking and response. For example, to promote reflection-in-action for learners who are at the novice or advanced beginner stages (Benner, 1984), a faculty member could be present in the patient care setting to guide the students' thoughts and actions at particular times. Lower level questioning could be interjected, such as the following: "I noticed you elevated the head of the bed (very good); explain the rationale behind your action." Or, to guide the student toward another action, the faculty member may ask, "Is there any other action you could initiate that would also help your patient's oxygenation status?"

A strategy combining the use of role modeling and thinking out loud could be used to demonstrate reflection-in-action across the spectrum of learning (Banning, 2008). Imagine students observing two faculty "thinking out loud" as they provide patient care. Faculty using this technique of reflection-in-action could role model critical thinking and reflective thinking as they demonstrate principles of prioritization, delegation, and communication. The complexity of the scenario would be designed and scripted to meet specific learning needs of the students. This learning experience should integrate a debriefing session to allow students time to recognize and reflect on their learning. Additional scenarios that require learners to provide patient care based on the same objectives could be developed and initiated by students immediately after the debriefing session to support their transfer of learning.

Numerous frameworks have been developed to assist faculty in the process of facilitating reflection-on-action. Johns (2004) describes the reflective cycle outlined by Gibbs in 1988, noting that it assists in the transfer of insight into practice through the use of questioning. Questions using the Gibbs' reflective cycle are posed, guiding the discussion by (a) beginning with a description of the event, "What happened?" (b) progressing to a discussion of feelings, "What were you thinking and feeling?" (c) evaluating the experience, "What was good and bad about the experience?" (d) engaging in analysis, "What sense can you make of the situation?"(e) performing a self-critique, "What else could you have done?" and (f) generating an action plan, "If it arose again, what would you do?" (p.17). Johns (1995) developed a model for structured reflection that provided cue questions based on Carper's four ways of knowing (Carper, 1978) to support the process of guided reflection. Carper's fundamental patterns of knowing in nursing include four fundamental, interrelated ways of knowing which allow for "an increased awareness of the complexity and diversity of nursing knowledge" (p. 21). The first way of knowing — empirical — is aimed at developing theoretical explanations. Empirical knowledge is knowledge that can be methodically organized into general laws and theories. The second way of knowing — aesthetics — can be traced to (Leddy, 2011) and is the difference between recognition and perception. The third way of knowing is personal knowledge and involves the relationships between patients and the nurse. Personal knowledge, according to Carper, is the most essential in understanding what health means to the individual. Ethics, the final way of knowing, represents the moral component and consists of professional obligations, norms, and ethical codes.

Utilizing the framework provided by Johns (2004), the facilitator poses questions to stimulate thinking in each of Carper's four ways of knowing and to stimulate thoughtful reflection. Examples include the following:

Empirical   "What knowledge informed or might have informed you?"

Aesthetic   "What particular issues seem significant to pay attention to?"

Personal   "What factors influenced the way you felt, thought or responded?"

Ethical   "To what extent did you act for the best and in tune with your values?"

Reflection   "How might you respond more effectively given this situation again?"

A modification to the model for structured reflection was derived from the outcome of a research study and input received from experts in grounded theory methodology. The Facilitator's Tool for Guided Reflection Sessions (see Table 7-2) was used in a pilot study that was part of the initial NLN/Laerdal Simulation Study. Findings revealed that students at the novice level used trial and error decision-making that demonstrated minimal knowledge transfer, and the patient care they planned was prioritized around the need to complete tasks (Decker, 2007).

Table 7-2 Facilitator's Tool for Guided Reflection Sessions	
Ways of Knowing	Open-ended Questions/Statements to Encourage Reflection-on-Action
Empirical	• Talk to me about the knowledge, skills, and experiences you have that helped you provide patient care during this simulated experience.
Aesthetic	• Talk to me about the problem your patient was having. • What was your main goal during this simulation?
Personal	• Tell me what influenced your actions during the scenario. • Talk to me about how this experience made you feel. • Talk to me about how satisfied you are with the actions you initiated during this scenario.
Ethical	• Talk to me about how your personal values and beliefs influenced your actions during this experience.
Reflection	• Talk to me about how you knew what to do during this situation. • What would you do differently if we went back into the patient's room and repeated the scenario right now? • Discuss how you will use what was learned in this experience in the future?

EVALUATING DEBRIEFING

Assessment of debriefing can involve evaluation of either the actual debriefing experience or its outcomes. There are several instruments available to look at the quality of the debriefing and a newer one that measures the participant experience of debriefing. Selection of an instrument to evaluate debriefing is dependent on the desired information and how the data will be used.

DASH©

The Debriefing Assessment for Simulation in Healthcare (DASH) and the long and short versions of the Debriefing Assessment for Simulation in Healthcare-Student Version© (DASH-SV) are instruments designed to rate the quality of debriefing. Because the elements of these instruments are based on the principles of debriefing, they can be used to evaluate many different types of methods and situations. The DASH is a tool designed to be used by peer-faculty while the DASH-SV is used by the debriefing participants; yet both evaluate the quality of debriefing. The two DASH–SV versions use the same six criteria and effectiveness scale as the DASH, but report the data from the student perspective. Criterion and content validity for the DASH have been established by the authors who, collectively, have 20 years experience debriefing medical students. All versions of the DASH instrument use a behaviorally anchored rating scale to identify the extent to which raters (faculty peers or students) perceive that the debriefing facilitator or instructor demonstrated six elements of effective debriefing following simulation experiences (Simon, Rudolph, & Raemer, 2009). Initial reliability of the DASH-SV was determined to be 0.82 (N = 6, M = 29.537, variance = 24.259, SD = 4.925) using a Cronbach's alpha analysis, and there was also good internal consistency between the items on the DASH and the DASH-SV (.89) supporting the assumption of unidimensionality of the tools (Dreifuerst, 2012).

The DASH and both versions of the DASH–SV use a seven-point effectiveness scale that is a "behaviorally anchored rating scale that describes and reflects the six key elements describing behaviors necessary to execute an effective debriefing" (Simon et al., 2009, p. 3) to document the debriefing assessment. Raters evaluate the ability of the debriefing facilitator to achieve the following elements:

- (The debriefer) Establishes an engaging learning environment.
- (The debriefer) Maintains an engaging learning environment.
- (The debriefer) Structures debriefing in an organized way.
- (The debriefer) Provokes engaging discussions.
- (The debriefer) Identifies and explores performance gaps.
- (The debriefer) Helps simulation participants achieve or sustain good practice.

(Simon et al., p. 3).

Elements are high-level concepts that describe a whole area or concept of debriefing behavior. Each element also includes dimensions that are used to describe parts of the element. Examples are also provided as further explanation for the rater using the tool. Raters score each element using their best judgment of the extent to which the debriefing facilitator demonstrated the element as a whole.

All versions of the DASH instrument have been used to assess debriefing in a variety of simulation settings with different types of health care students at different levels of educational preparation. It adapts well. However, consistent inter-rater reliability is dependent on the training the rater receives; therefore regular training sessions are offered by the authors of the instrument (Simon et al., 2009).

Debriefing Experience Scale (DES)

Another instrument for evaluating debriefing is the Debriefing Experience Scale (DES) developed by Reed (2012). The DES is a newer tool for students and participants to use for evaluating debriefing. The following two concepts are measured: the student experience during debriefing and the importance of those experiences. The Experience Scale portion of the DES uses a Likert-type scale rating of 1 (strongly disagree) to 5 (strongly agree) and the Importance Scale portion of the DES uses a Likert-type scale rating of 1 (not important) to 5 (very important) to measure student responses to the same 20 items on the instrument (Reed, 2012). The items on the instrument are organized into four subscales:

1. Analyzing Thoughts and Feelings

2. Learning and Making Connections

3. Facilitator Skill in Conducting Debriefing

4. Appropriate Facilitator Guidance (Reed, p. e5)

Experience is important to measure because it reflects how the participant felt and perceived the debriefing went. Importance on the other hand reflects how critical the participant perceives the item to be related to their debriefing experience. Since both concepts impact learning and overall engagement in the process, understanding this information could inform future debriefing strategies and outcomes.

The instrument demonstrated high reliability using Cronbach's Alpha analysis with both the Experience Scale (.93) and the Importance Scale (.91) when used with pre-licensure nursing students in studies comparing their experiences with different debriefing types that use a facilitator. This debriefing evaluation instrument could be used with other types of health care professionals, though reliability testing would be suggested.

Both the DASH and the DES provide opportunities for evaluating the debriefing experience. This is an important consideration when looking at learning as an outcome or as an educational quality measure. (Note: The authors acknowledge Shelly Reed, DNP, RN, for her contribution to this section.)

SPECIAL DEBRIEFING CIRCUMSTANCES

Debriefing can occur in different ways. While group interaction and discussion involving the debriefing facilitator and the participants in the simulation experience is most common, other options exist. These can be particularly useful when there are special circumstances that can impact debriefing group interaction. Some of those include a variation in the number of students being debriefed, the educational framework and experience the student comes with, the format for the debriefing, and the impact of strong emotions.

DEBRIEFING INTERPROFESSIONAL TEAMS

Research has demonstrated that working together as an interdisciplinary team decreases costs, prevents mistakes, promotes patient safety, and improves patient satisfaction (Allen, Penn, & Nora, 2006; Institute of Medicine, 2011). As a member of the health care team, each individual is expected to promote safe, quality patient care through interprofessional collaboration, communication, and coordination. Preparing health professions to function competently in this collegial environment requires a transformation in the current educational process (Benner et al., 2010). Shapiro and colleagues (2008) also stressed that knowing about teamwork does not guarantee an individual is able to demonstrate the knowledge, skills, behaviors, and attitudes required to participate as a member of an interprofessional team. Simulation provides a unique tool to teach and assess teamwork in a challenging, psychologically safe environment.

Team training endeavors require methodical preparation, implementation, and evaluation. Little research is available to determine best practices for debriefing interprofessional teams. Individuals facilitating interprofessional team debriefings do, however, need to be competent in debriefing skills and expand these to include techniques that elicit team interaction. Faculty from all disciplines represented need to be present at these debriefings to convey the importance of the learning activity to the learner. A modification of the Plus Delta technique in which team members discuss "what went well," "what did not go well, and what could have been better" was conducted by Miller, Riley, Davis, and Hansen (2008) and interprofessional team members. Facilitators used video playback to highlight and promote discussion of both positive teamwork and communication lapses that occurred during scenarios.

Debriefing guidelines provided through TeamSTEPPS (Agency for Healthcare Research and Quality, 2006) stress the importance of centering discussion on team performance. TeamSTEPPS also presents a modification of the Alpha Delta format that encourages the team to analyze "why the event occurred, what worked and what did not work" (p. 15). The goal of an interprofessional debriefing is to provide a supportive environment where all participants are respected and feel free to verbalize in a truthful manner. Guidelines to assist in facilitating these discussions include many strategies to promote teamwork (Table 7-2).

Table 7-3 Interprofessional Team Debriefing

Facilitation Guideline for Debriefing Interprofessional Teams
• Clarify the objectives of the debrief specific to team performance.
• Maintain the discussion "team-centered."
• Vary the facilitation to meet the needs of the various team members.
• Allow team members to speak. Don't interrupt.
• Promote team self-discovery.
• Use Socratic questioning to promote discussion.
• Redirect questions back to the team. Encourage team members to discover their own answers.
• Involve quiet team members.
• Encourage team members to talk among themselves.
• Ask the team to discuss factors that promoted or impeded their success.
• Promote transfer of the activity's objectives to patient care.
• Use active listening.
• Include video strategically to stimulate discussion.
• Briefly summarize the debrief, highlighting the objectives.

(McDonnell, Jobe, & Dismukes, 1997)

DEBRIEFING LARGE GROUPS

There are situations when debriefing involves a large group of participants. This can provide unique challenges for the facilitator. Engaging learners and keeping them actively involved in the debriefing process can be difficult with a large group. Because of this, debriefing a large group may start out with everyone together or it may be divided into small subgroups from the start or later in the debriefing process. Either way, each subgroup would need its own facilitator to promote learner participation. After the initial debrief, subgroups could reconvene allowing a designated leader from each groups to provide a summary of their discussion (Fanning & Gaba, 2007).

WRITTEN DEBRIEFING

Another form of debriefing that has been used with both simulated and actual clinical experiences is written debriefing. An advantage to written debriefing is the recording that can be accessed later to assist in recollection of the experience or the key elements of debriefing. In fact, it has been suggested that written debriefing can be more reflective than verbal, therefore facilitating better learning (Petranek, 2000), although this continues to be debated (Kuiper, 2005).

Written debriefing can include reflective journaling techniques and a diary of events. Journaling can prompt personal reflection and reframing of the experience through meta-cognition. This also occurs in oral debriefing. However, the time involved in journaling and reflection can be more substantial, leading to deeper processing and self-regulation (Kuiper, 2004). Moreover, journals can be used as a form of communication between students and faculty about the clinical experience in a form of dialog where the instructor responds to the student or prompts further reflection and learning.

In an age of technology and rapid interaction, written debriefing can also be done through blogging, texting, or posting through social networking using mobile devices (Skiba, 2011). Each of these is a form of an online interactive diary or journal that might be more particularly appealing to students who are savvy with technology and prefer instant communication with peers and debriefing facilitators.

The most critical factor with written debriefing is facilitator feedback to what is written by the participants. Feedback should be specific to the objectives for the simulation or clinical experience and the participant's reflection and written thoughts. Feedback should be timely and constructive.

Online Debriefing

Strategies identified to support individual reflection other than written journal writing include audio- or videotaped journaling (Kuiper, 2005), email-based dialogues (Henderson & Johnson, 2002), and blogs (Thomas, Bertram, & Allen, 2012). The use of these online strategies has been shown to enhance the learner's feelings of self-awareness, self-confidence, and critical reasoning and reflective thought. When group activities are integrated into the experiences, learners are able to view different perspectives and provide peers with constructive critiques (Carkhuff, 1996; Westberg & Jason, 2001). Thomas et al. explored the use of a teaching-learning simulation blog to facilitate reflective thought by creating a virtual registered nurse who transitioned from new graduate through her first year of practice. Students who participated in the experience felt the experience promoted critical thinking and communication skills.

Debriefing the Devastating Incident or Poor Performance

Sometimes the simulation involves a very emotionally difficult scenario, a devastating incident, or a poor student performance. These instances can bring about a highly emotional debriefing experience that can be focused on the release of emotions or the correction of behavior. When this occurs, the debriefing process engaged by the facilitator can be critical to achieving the intended outcome of the debriefing.

Performance refers to the actual behaviors enacted by a team or individuals involved in the simulation or clinical experience. Evaluation is the comparison of actions, decisions, and outcomes demonstrated in the simulation or clinical experience with what was intended or expected (Rosen et al., 2010). One of the benefits of using simulated patients is that poor performance does not necessarily result in harm; therefore it is often considered a safe environment. A poor performance can, however, be devastating to the participants in the experience. Allowing an emotional release can be initially effective; however, including time in debriefing for assessment and correction of the errors in decisions, behaviors, and judgment is also important (Rudolph et al., 2008). If the debriefing continues to focus on the emotional release without a review of why the poor performance occurred and how to change it, then learning does not occur and behavior will not change the next time this clinical situation is encountered. Therefore it is important to allow debriefing time for both (Arafeh et al., 2010; Cantrell, 2008; Dreifuerst, 2009; Flannagan, 2008). While the use of constructive feedback is always advised, it is particularly important when there has been a poor performance or negative patient outcome. This does not mean that critical judgment is avoided, but it should be delivered respectfully and in a manner that maintains simulation as a safe learning environment (Rudolph, Simon, Dufresne, & Raemer, 2006).

This is also true for the devastating scenario experience. Given the fidelity of simulation and the association with critical human experiences, it is not unusual for a participant to encounter a simulation that mirrors a life experience in a way that triggers an emotional response. Likewise, the participants can develop an emotional tie to the simulated patient that is reflected in emotions like crying or anger related to what was experienced. When these occur, it is also important for the facilitator to acknowledge the emotion and solicit discussion about it initially. However, this too is a situation that can result in the entire debriefing being focused on emotion rather than on solidifying the learning. Therefore, the facilitator needs to balance the time spent on emotional release with the reflective review of the actions, decisions, and outcomes of the experience to facilitate learning.

CONCLUSION

Debriefing and reflection are essential components of clinical learning in practice settings and simulation environments (Dreifuerst, 2009; Shinnick et al., 2011). Revisiting the clinical events to understand the participant's behaviors, decision-making, and the impact on patient outcomes solidifies learning from the experience. There are many debriefing methods that can be used to guide the reflective process. Each method, however, takes into account the best practices in debriefing regarding timing, environment, the use of constructive critique, and respect for all participants.

Debriefing should manifest the objectives of the clinical experience and recall the events of the simulation. A facilitator can be very effective to guide reflection and manage the experience; however, peer and self-debriefing are also valuable for many learners. Evaluating debriefing is also important for understanding its impact on learners and to foster improvement in facilitators and methods. There is a need for continued research into best debriefing practices that will engage participants, foster learning that can transfer to other settings, and result in improved clinical outcomes.

REFERENCES

Adler, A. B., Castro, C. A., & McGurk, D. (2009). Time-driven battlemind psychological debriefing: A group-level early intervention in combat. *Military Medicine, 174*(1), 21-28.

Agency for Healthcare Research and Quality. (2006). Leadership. *In Instructor Guide: TeamSTEPPS Team Strategies & Tools to Enhance Performance & Patient Safety* (pp.1-24). Washington, DC: Author.

Allen, D. D., Penn, M. A., & Nora, L. M. (2006). Interdisciplinary healthcare education: Fact of fiction? *American Journal of Pharmaceutical Education, 70*(2), 1-2.

American Heart Association (2010). Structured and supported debriefing. In http://npsc.us/ acls/structured-and-supported-debriefing-aha?device=desktop. Retrieved July 5, 2012 from http://npsc.us/acls/structured-and-supported-debriefing-aha?device=desktop

Arafeh, J. M., Hansen, S. S., & Nichols, A. (2010). Debriefing in simulated-based learning: Facilitating a reflective discussion. *Journal of Perinatal & Neonatal Nursing, 24*(4), 302-309.

Banning, M. (2008). The think aloud approach as an educational tool to develop and assess clinical reasoning in undergraduate students. *Nurse Education Today, 28*(1), 8-14.

Benner, P. (1984). *From novice to expert: Excellence and power in clinical nursing practice.* Menlo Park, CA: Addison-Wesley. Benner, P., Sutphen, M., Leonard, V., & Day, L. (2010). Educating nurses: Acall for radical transformation. SanFrancisco: Jossey-Bass.

Bybee, R. W., Buchwald, C. E., Crissman, S., Heil, D. R., Kuebis, P. J., Matsumoto, C., & McInerney, J. D. (1989). *Science and technology education for the elementary years: Frameworks for curriculum and instruction.* Washington, DC: National Center for Improving Science Education.

Cantrell, M. A. (2008). The importance of debriefing in clinical simulations. *Clinical Simulation in Nursing, 4*(2), e19-e23. doi:10.1016/j.ecns.2008.06.006

Caputi, L., & Engelmann, L. (2007). *Teaching nursing: The art and science* (2nd ed., Vol. 1). Glen Ellyn, IL: College of DuPage Press.

Carkhuff, M. H. (1996). Reflective learning: Work groups as learning groups. *Journal of Continuing Education in Nursing, 27*(5), 209-214.

Carper, B. A. (1978). Fundamental patterns of knowing in nursing. *Advances in Nursing Sciences, 1*, 13-23.

Decker, S. (2007). Integrating guided reflection into simulated learning experiences. In P. Jeffries (Ed.), *Simulation in nursing* (pp. 21–33). New York, NY: National League for Nursing.

Decker, S., Gore, T. T., & Feken, C. (2011). Simulation. In T. J. Bristol & J. Zerwekh (Eds.), *Essentials of e-learning for nurse educators* (pp. 277-294). Philadelphia, PA: F. A. Davis Company.

Dieckmann, P., Friis, S. M., Lippert, A., & Ostergaard, D. (2009). The art and science of debriefing in simulation: Ideal and practice. *Medical Teacher, 31*, e287-e294

Dismukes, R. K., Gaba, D. M., & Howard, S. K. (2006). So many roads: Facilitated debriefing in health care. *Simulation in Healthcare, 1*(1), 23–25.

Dreifuerst, K. T. (2009). The essentials of debriefing in simulation learning: A concept analysis. *Nursing Education Perspectives, 30*(2), 109–114.

Dreifuerst, K. T. (2010). *Debriefing for meaningful learning: Fostering development of clinical reasoning through simulation* (Doctoral dissertation). Retrieved from http://hdl. handle.net/1805/2459

Dreifuerst, K. T. (2012, in press). Using debriefing for meaningful learning to foster development of clinical reasoning in simulation. *Journal of Nursing Education, 51*(6).

Fanning, R. M., & Gaba, D. M. (2007). The role of debriefing in simulation-based learning. *Simulation in Healthcare, 2*(2), 115-125.

Flannagan, B. (2008). Debriefing: Theory and techniques. In R. H. Riley (Ed.), *Manual of simulation in healthcare* (pp. 155-170). New York, NY: Oxford University Press.

Henderson, .P, Johnson, M. (2002). Assisting medical students to conduct empathic conversations with patients in a sexual medical clinic. *Sexually Transmitted Infections, 78*(4), 246-249.

Institute of Medicine. (2011). *The future of nursing leading change, advancing health.* Washington, DC: National Academies Press.

Jeffries, P. R. (2005). A framework for designing, implementing, and evaluating simulations used as teaching strategies in nursing. *Nursing Education Perspectives, 26*(2), 96-103.

Jeffries, P. R., & Rizzolo, M. A. (2006). Designing and implementing models for the innovative use of simulation to teach nursing care of ill adults and children: A national, multi-site, multi-method study. *National League for Nursing and Laerdal research year two — end of year report.* Retrieved July 5, 2012, from http://www.nln.org/research. LaerdalY2End.pdf

Johns, C. (1995). Framing learning through reflection within Carper's fundamental ways of knowing in nursing. *Journal of Advanced Nursing, 22*(2), 226-234.

Johns, C. (2004). *Becoming a reflective practitioner* (2nd ed.). Malden, MA: Blackwell.

Kuiper, R. (2005). Self-regulated learning during a clinical preceptorship: The reflections of senior baccalaureate nursing students. *Nursing Education Perspectives, 26*(6), 351-356.

Lasater, K. (2007). High-fidelity simulation and the development of clinical judgment: Students' experiences. *Journal of Nursing Education, 46*(6), 269-276.

Leddy, Tom, "Dewey's Aesthetics", The Stanford Encyclopedia of Philosophy (Winter 2011 Edition), Edward N. Zalta (ed.),http://plato.stanford.edu/archives/win2011/entries/dewey-aesthetics/>. Retrieved July 5, 2012.

McDonnell, L. K., Jobe, K. K., & Dismukes, R. K. (1997). Facilitating LOS debriefings: A training manual. *Flight Safety Digest, 16*(11), 1-24.

McGaghie, W. C., Issenberg, S. B., Petrusa, E. R., & Scalese, R. J. (2010). A critical review of simulation-based medical education research: 2003-2009. *Medical Education, 44*(1), 50-63. doi:10.1111/j.1365-2923.2009.03547.x

Miller, K. K., Riley, W., Davis, S., & Hansen, H. E. (2008). In situ simulation a method of experiential learning to promote safety and team behavior. *Journal of Perinatal Neonatal Nursing, 22*(2), 105-113.

Overstreet, M. (2010). E-chats: The seven components of nursing debriefing. The Journal of Continuing *Education in Nursing, 41*(12), 538-539.

Petranek, C. F. (2000). Written debriefing: The next vital step in learning withsimulations. *Simulation & Gaming, 31*, 108-118.

Raemer, D., Anderson, M., Cheng, A., Fanning, R., Nadkarni, V., & Savoldelli, G. (2011). Research regarding debriefing as part of the learning process. *Simulation in Healthcare, 6*(7), 552-557.

Reed, S. J. (in press). Debriefing experience scale: Development of a tool to evaluate the student learning experience in debriefing. *Clinical Simulation in Nursing, 8*(7). doi:10.1016/j.ecns.2011.11.002

Regehr, C. (2001). Crisis debriefing groups for emergency responders: Reviewing the evidence. *Brief Treatment and Crisis Intervention, 1*(2), 87-100.

Rosen, M., Weaver, S., Lazzara, E., Salas, E., Wu, T., Silvestri, S., . . . King, H. (2010). Tools for evaluating team performance in simulation-based training. *Journal of Emergencies, Trauma and Shock, 3*(4), 353-359. doi:10.4103/0974-2700.70746

Rudolph, J. W., Simon, R., Dufresne, R. L., & Raemer, D. B. (2006). There's no such thing as "nonjudgmental" debriefing: A theory and method for debriefing with good judgment. *Simulation in Healthcare, 1*, 49-55.

Rudolph, J. W., Simon, R., Raemer, D. B., & Eppich, W. J. (2008). Debriefing as formative assessment: Closing performance gaps in medical education. *Academic Emergency Medicine, 15*(11), 1010-1016. doi:10.1111/j.1553-2712.2008.00248.x

Rudolph, J. W., Simon, R., Rivard, P., Dufresne, R. L., & Raemer, D. B. (2007). Debriefing with good judgment: Combining rigorous feedback with genuine inquiry. *Anesthesiology Clinics, 25*(2), 361-376.

Schön, D. A. (1983). *The reflective practitioner: How professionals think in action.* New York, NY: Basic Books.

Seaman, D. F., & Fellenz, R. A. (1989). *Effective strategies for teaching adults.* Columbus, OH: Merrill.

Shapiro, M. J., Gardner, R., Godwin, S. A., Jay, G. D., Lindquist, D. G., Salisbury, M. L., & Salas, E. (2008). Defining team performance for simulation-based training: Methodology, metrics, and opportunities for Emergency Medicine. *Academic Emergency Medicine, 15* (11), 1088-1097. doi:10.1111/j.1553-2712.2008.00251.x

Shinnick, M. A., Woo, M. A., & Mentes, J. C. (2011). Human patient simulation: State of the science in prelicensure nursing education. *Journal of Nursing Education, 50*(2), 65-72. doi:10.3928/01484834-20101230-01

Simon, R., Rudolph, J. W., & Raemer, D. B. (2009). Debriefing assessment for simulation in health care© — student version. *In Center for Medical Simulation.* Retrieved July 5, 2012, from http://www.harvardmedsim.org/debriefing-assesment-simulation-health care.php

Skiba, D. J. (2011). On the horizon mobile devices: Are they a distraction or another learning tool? *Nursing Education Perspectives, 32*(3), 195-197.

Tanner, C. A. (2006). Thinking like a nurse: A research-based model of clinical judgment in nursing. *Journal of Nursing Education, 45*(6), 204-211.

Thomas, C. M., Bertram, E., & Allen, R. (2012). Preparing for transition to professional practice: Creating a simulated blog and reflective journaling activity. *Clinical Simulation in Nursing, 8,* e87-e95. doi:10.1016/j.ecns.2010.07.004

Van Heukelom, J. N., Begaz, T., Treat, R., (2010). Comparison of post simulation debriefing versus in-simulation debriefing in medical simulation. *Simulation in Healthcare, 5*(2), 91-97.

Westberg, J., & Jason, H. (2001). *Fostering reflection and providing feedback.* New York, NY: Springer Publishing.

Wickers, M. P. (2010). Establishing the climate for a successful debriefing. *Clinical Simulations in Nursing, 6,* e83-e86.

Wotton, K., Davis, J., Button, D., Kelton, M. (2010). Third-year undergraduate nursing students' perceptions of high-fidelity simulation. *Journal of Nursing Education, 49*(11), 632-639. doi:10.3928/014834-20100831-01

CHAPTER 8
EVALUATION: A CRITICAL STEP IN SIMULATION PRACTICE AND RESEARCH

Katie Anne Adamson, PhD, RN
Pamela R. Jeffries, PhD, RN, FAAN, ANEF
Kristen J. Rogers, MSN, RN

"How to tell students what to look for

without telling them what to see is the

dilemma of teaching."

–Lascelles Abercrombie

EVALUATION: A CRITICAL STEP IN SIMULATION PRACTICE AND RESEARCH

Evaluation is a critical and often overlooked component of simulation practice and research (Diekelmann & Ironside, 2002). While the literature is exploding with new instruments and strategies for simulation evaluation, the practical application of such work can be daunting. Nurse educators face the challenge of selecting appropriate evaluation strategies both to examine the design and implementation of the simulation activity itself and to assess learning outcomes from the simulation activity (Campbell, 2010). Each of these areas of evaluation is complex and may include both formative and summative components. This chapter will present a basic, systematic process for simulation evaluation, a summary of selected types of evaluation instruments, and an overview of simulation evaluation strategies that may be implemented at various phases of the simulation process. Finally, the chapter will conclude with a review of issues related to evaluation, including assessing the validity and reliability of simulation evaluation data.

BASICS OF EVALUATION: A SYSTEMATIC PROCESS

Simulation evaluation is a systematic process that includes a number of specific steps. However, the educator's philosophy about simulation will influence frequency and timing of evaluations, methods, and how results are interpreted and used (Bourke & Ihrke, 2005). The basic steps in the process of simulation evaluation include the following: (a) identifying the purpose of the evaluation; (b) determining a timeframe for the evaluation; (c) identifying when to evaluate; (d) developing an evaluation plan; (e) selecting the evaluation instrument(s); (f) collecting data; and (g) interpreting the data (Billings & Halstead, 2005). The following sections describe each of these steps as they relate to simulation evaluation.

Identifying the Purpose of the Evaluation

After identifying the need for an evaluation, the first and most important step is to identify the purpose of the evaluation. One can achieve clarity about what is being evaluated by articulating the questions that the evaluation data will answer. The questions can be focused, such as whether students can perform a selected skill set or care for a specific type of client, or the questions may be broad and encompassing, for example, whether there is a higher order of thinking involved when students are immersed in a teaching-learning environment using simulations. Additionally, the purpose of an evaluation may be to provide information about the instructional design of the simulation itself; the educational practices incorporated in the simulation to promote learning; timing; clarity of the simulation; or the overall flow and fidelity of the simulation. In all cases, the purpose of the evaluation should be clear to students, faculty, and all involved. Involving all parties, especially learners, early in the evaluation process helps them see how well the objectives of the course have been met, in addition to identifying their own strengths, areas for improvement, and competency level.

Determining a Timeframe to Evaluate

The timeframe for evaluation is partly determined by whether the purpose of the evaluation is to provide formative or summative feedback. Summative evaluations focus on goal attainment and provide feedback about a completed simulation or at the end of a learning period to identify what has been learned or accomplished (Gaberson & Oermann, 2010). In contrast, formative evaluations focus on progress toward goal attainment and can contribute to self-reflection and help identify areas for future improvement (Oermann & Gaberson, 2006; Gaberson & Oermann). Formative evaluations typically take place at a point before the end of a course or learning experience and assess a particular teaching-learning activity, instruction, or scenario. Both summative and formative evaluations may be helpful in examining all stages of simulation design, implementation, and outcomes and may include a variety of data collection methods.

When assessing learning outcomes, summative evaluation may include using a simulation to assess students' competence on selected critical behaviors, skills, and knowledge at the end of the course. The focus is on a whole event or concept area for which outcomes need to be measured. Measured outcomes may involve a grade or a pass/fail judgment, and they may entail remediation if this is a required competency that students need before progressing on in the course or curriculum. Formative evaluation may include using simulation to assess students as they progress through a course to provide feedback that will help them improve and perform better on future formative or summative evaluations. Likewise, both summative and formative evaluations may be used to assess the design and implementation of simulations. A summative evaluation of the design or implementation of a simulation may be completed during the development or piloting of a simulation while a formative evaluation would be completed to reflect on the quality of a completed simulation.

Identifying When to Evaluate

Determining when to evaluate also depends on whether the simulation evaluation is formative or summative. If formative, the evaluation occurs after the students have participated in the simulation activity, but while there is still time in the course for them to strengthen their weak areas and improve their performance if they did not meet expectations. If summative, most likely for a grade or to document a specific competency level before the learner can progress, the evaluation typically occurs at the end of the course or at the end of a module or component of instruction.

Developing an Evaluation Plan

When implementing simulations or any other type of innovative teaching strategy, an evaluation plan should be developed, as mentioned, to ensure that the strategy is effective and that students are indeed learning from the activity. The plan needs to include the specific type of evaluation to be carried out, procedures detailing exactly how the evaluation will be conducted, identification of who will do it, instruments or tools to be used, and the intended outcomes or activities to be evaluated. When several educators are involved in the course, evaluation planning needs to include all of them. As the last, and very important, component in the teaching-learning process, a well-organized evaluation can be implemented more easily if all components have been defined and prepared before the evaluation actually occurs.

Selecting the Evaluation Instrument(s)

Once the initial pieces of the evaluation plan are in place and the variables to be measured are clearly defined, the next step is to select or develop appropriate measurement instruments. The simulation literature is full of evaluation instruments for assessing various components of simulation design, implementation, and outcomes, and each has its own strengths and weaknesses. Several reviews from the literature may be helpful for educators selecting simulation evaluation instruments:

(a) Davis and Kimble (2011) reviewed six rubrics from the literature that have been developed to evaluate students based on the 2008 Baccalaureate Essentials. Their review provides details about the psychometric characteristics of each instrument, as well as what learning domains and which essentials each instrument is designed to evaluate.

(b) Kardong-Edgren, Adamson, and Fitzgerald (2010 completed a review of various types of simulation evaluation instruments available in the literature. The review is organized according to the learning domain the instruments are designed to evaluate (cognitive, psychomotor, or affective) and includes sections about instruments designed to measure elements of team performance, as well as instruments in development.

(c) Kogan, Holmboe, and Hauer (2009) completed a review of instruments designed to evaluate clinical skills of medical trainees. This review includes descriptions of 55 instruments from the literature and provides useful data about the structure and validity of each.

Depending upon the purpose of the evaluation, educators may choose to use questionnaires, observations, checklists, attitude scales, journals, diaries, anecdotal notes, or other types of evaluation instruments. In any case, it is important to have information about the reliability and validity of data produced using the instruments that can help guide the implementation of the instrument and interpretation of the data produced.

Questionnaires

Questionnaires are widely used to evaluate simulation design, implementation, and outcomes. Data gathered using questionnaires is typically self-reported by the learner, and items need to be concise, clear, and simple so the respondents can understand what is being asked (Polit & Hungler, 1995). Examples of questionnaires used to evaluate the design and implementation of simulations include the Simulation Design Scale and the Educational Practices in Simulation Scale (Jeffries et.al, 2004). Examples of questionnaires used to evaluate outcomes from simulation range from measures of student satisfaction and confidence such as the Student Satisfaction and Self Confidence in Learning Instruments (National League for Nursing, 2005) and the Emergency Response Confidence Tool (Arnold et al., 2009), to students' perceptions of the simulated clinical activity (Robertson, 2006), to measures of basic knowledge (Hoffman, O'Donnell, & Kim, 2007; Lewis & Ciak, 2011), Health-Education Systems, Inc. (HESI)-type exams (Howard, Ross, Mitchell, & Nelson, 2010), and critical thinking assessments (Chau et al., 2001; Ravert, 2008). Questionnaires may also be used to allow students to reflect on their own performance and evaluate the use of simulation in preparing students for clinical practice and transition to practice (McCaughey & Traynor, 2010).

Observation and checklists

Observation-based evaluations involve an evaluator, typically an instructor or another trained participant, observing skills or critical behaviors of students while they participate in the simulation. Observation or a performance appraisal is useful for evaluating skill performance, skill competency, development of selected values and attitudes, and communication skills. Ideally, students are provided feedback about what has been observed immediately after the simulated event in the debriefing or guided reflection period that follows the simulation itself. In formative evaluations, informing students immediately after the behavior allows time for remediation and correction of any incorrect activity or skill. For summative evaluations, an evaluator other than the student's instructor should complete the observation-based evaluation. This minimizes the potential for bias, halo-effects, or other confounding variables that may interfere with an objective, observation-based evaluation.

Various components of students' performance may be observed and evaluated during a simulation. Observation-based evaluation instruments from the literature include tools to assess communication skills (Klackovich & Dela Cruz, 2006), teamwork and crew resource management skills (Malec et al., 2007), and advanced technical skills (e.g., airway management) (Morgan & Cleave-Hogg, 2000). Additionally, instruments are used to evaluate broader behaviors such as clinical judgment abilities (Lasater, 2007) or the demonstration of the Baccalaureate Essentials (Todd, Manz, Hawkins, Parsons, & Hercinger, 2008). One caveat related to observation-based evaluation instruments is that the behavior or skill that is being assessed must be carefully built into the simulation to allow students to demonstrate it and be evaluated on it. For example, a student may not be fairly evaluated on his or her clinical judgment abilities during a scenario that is designed to practice or demonstrate a straight-forward skill. Evaluators must have adequate training using observation-based evaluation instruments, and if more than one rater is going to complete the evaluations, close attention must be paid to inter-rater reliability of ratings.

Checklists, a subset of observation-based evaluation instruments, are often are used to evaluate an expected student behavior during simulation activities. Specifically, checklists indicate that the behavior has been met or not. Weighted checklists may also be designed so that a scoring mechanism is included for each item, giving more important behaviors on the checklist more weight (e.g., two points instead of one point). This type of instrument is helpful for both formative and summative evaluation. Checklists are easy to complete and can be used for many purposes, such as assessing skill performance outcomes in the psychomotor realm. If the learning outcome relates to performance of a beginning skill (e.g., catheterization), the educator, using a checklist, clarifies for the learner the steps or the required performance criteria. Common checklists found in the literature include CPR Critical Skills Testing Checklist for Basic Life Support (BLS) training and Megacode Testing Checklists for Advanced Cardiac Life Support (ACLS) training (American Heart Association, 2011).

When simulation activities are video-recorded, observation-based evaluations, including checklists, may be used to provide learners with an opportunity to assess their own performance (Billings & Halstead, 2005). This practice also provides educators flexibility regarding when and where they evaluate learners. For example, the tape can be reviewed in the faculty member's office at a later time. In one study, Winters, Hauck, Riggs, Clawson, and Collins (2003) found that videotaping skill performance was positive for students and instructors alike; students report increased confidence when performing skills in the clinical setting after reviewing their videotaped performance along with the instructor, and faculty reported improvement in students' abilities to perform the videotaped skills in the clinical setting. Overall, there is little evidence on best practices for using videotaping for debriefing; more research is needed in this pedagogical area.

Attitude scales

This type of instrument allows the educator to measure how the student feels about a particular subject or teaching and learning strategy such as simulation. These measures typically have Likert-like scales reflecting ranges from strongly agree to strongly disagree. Several types of attitude scales are used in simulation evaluation, such as measures of self-efficacy and satisfaction with the strategy as a method of instruction. Jeffries, Woolf, and Linde (2003) provide one example from the literature of using a Likert-like attitude scale to allow students to rate various aspects of an interactive simulated experience and a traditional learning experience.

Journal or diary

Journaling is a type of self-reporting students can do that is a narrative of their reflections, activities, and feelings about the performance. Journals can be a one-time assignment or a continuous evaluation method throughout the course or clinical experience so the educator can track reflections and experiences across time. The value of these tools depend on how they are planned, constructed, and used (Bourke & Ihrke, 2005). Marchigiano, Eduljee, and Harvey (2011) found that journaling enhanced students' thinking skills. Jenkins and Turick-Gibson (1999) used student journals to measure critical thinking when using simulations. Weller (2004) used thematic analysis of students' written comments when studying 33 fourth-year medical students to evaluate the use of simulation-based teaching in the context of management.

Anecdotal notes

This type of student evaluation with simulation is also described in the literature (Hample, Herbold, Schneider, & Sheeley, 1999; Jenkins & Turick-Gibson, 1999; Peterson & Bechtel, 2000). Anecdotal notes are narrative descriptions of the student's performance or behavior after an observed event (e.g., a simulation activity). Anecdotal notes are typically used in formative evaluations and their usefulness can be enhanced when clear objectives are identified in advance. Notations should be reviewed with the learner and may include learner feedback. This review with the learner helps identify opportunities for improvement (Gaberson & Oermann, 2010). Anecdotal notes are more valuable when they are collected over time, summarized, and assessed for patterns and trends. A continuous assessment of the learner decreases one-time biases and reflects a more fair judgment of the student or event. Trends may also be considered for summative evaluations.

Collecting Data

The purpose of the evaluation, including whether it is summative or formative, will determine how one will collect the data and the time needed to do the task. Various factors should be considered when collecting the data, including: data source, amount of data being collected, timing of the data collection, and whether the data collection is informal or formal. Informal data collecting includes spontaneous remarks from students that educators then use to draw conclusions about satisfaction with and learning from the event. In other cases, a formalized evaluation process takes place in which structured evaluation tools are used at a specific time. Timing of the data collection depends on the number of variables being assessed, and caution should be taken not to overburden students with data collection because results can be affected by this factor.

Interpreting the Data

In this step, the evaluation responses are interpreted to answer the evaluation questions that were asked before the process was implemented. Data must be put in a usable form so educators can understand their meaning and implications. Data interpretation should consider the context of the evaluation process, the frame of reference, objectivity, and legal and ethical issues (Billings & Halstead, 2005).

LEVELS OF EVALUATION IN SIMULATION AT THE PRE-IMPLEMENTATION, IMPLEMENTATION, AND OUTCOMES PHASES

Simulations can be evaluated at various phases and on several levels. Prior to implementing a simulation, educators may evaluate the design of the simulation and ensure that key features are adequately imbedded in the simulation. During the implementation phase, educators may evaluate how well evidence-based educational practices were demonstrated throughout the simulation activity. Finally, educators often want to evaluate learning outcomes from simulation activities. Kirkpatrick (1994) suggested four levels for evaluating outcomes from teaching and learning strategies such as simulation. These include: (a) the student's **reaction** to the simulation activity, (b) the student's **learning** from the simulation, (c) changes in the student's **behavior** as a result of the activity, and (d) the longer term **results** in practice that take place because of the activity. The following sections will review strategies for simulation evaluation on each of these levels — from pre-implementation through outcome evaluation.

Simulation Evaluation During the Pre-implementation Phase

To evaluate the design and development of a simulation that is created by nurse educators, Jeffries et al. (2004) developed the Simulation Design Scale (SDS) (see Table 8-1). The purpose of this tool is to provide the educator with feedback that can be utilized to improve the simulation design and implementation. The SDS provides measures of the importance of each design feature of the simulation in addition to the degree each design feature is adequately embedded within the simulation design.

Table 8-1 Simulation Design Scale (SDS): Components

Component	Description
Objectives/ Information	Clear objectives and time frame for the simulation are needed by students before the simulation begins. Information needs to be provided on what learners need to know and what they are expected to learn.
Student Support	Student support is offered before, during, and after a simulation.
	Support includes providing information and direction to the student prior to the simulation. During the simulation, cues can be provided to the students participating in the simulation via a lab test, a chest x-ray (CXR) report, a phone call from a physician or a nurse manager, or in other ways. After a simulation, support is provided during the debriefing. Students find the debriefing part of the simulation a most important aspect; instructors are helpful when they correct misinformation or inappropriate actions that happened in the scenario, in addition to emphasizing components that should have been done but were not or areas of nursing care that were done well.
Problem Solving/ Complexity	The simulation needs to be designed with problem solving components embedded in the scenario or case that is written. The level of problem solving needs to be considered (e.g., simple tasks and decisions if students are in a fundamentals course versus more complex problem solving if students are in an upper-level course and six months from graduating).
Fidelity	A simulation should be designed to be as close an approximation as possible to the real event or activity that is being developed to promote learning. Barrow and Feltovich (1987) suggest that the structure of a realistic, simulated clinical situation requires the following three elements:
	1) relatively little information should be available initially; 2) students should be allowed to investigate freely, employing questions in any sequence; and 3) students get important clinical information over time during the simulation.
Guided Reflection/ Debriefing	Guided reflection reinforces the positive aspects of the experience and encourages reflective learning, which allows the participant to link theory to practice and research, think critically, and discuss how to intervene professionally in complex situations (Bruce, Bridges, & Holcomb, 2003; Jenkins & Turick-Gibson, 1999; Jones, Cason, & Mancini, 2002; Thomas, O'Connor, Albert, Boutain, & Brandt, 2001; Rauen, 2001).
	At the end of the session, the group should discuss the process, outcome, and application of the scenario to clinical practice and review the relevant teaching points (Rauen, 2001). Jenkins and Turick-Gibson discuss how the last step in their simulation activity was to share and generalize information with the students.

The Simulation Design Scale (SDS) is a 20-item tool with subscales measuring various design features. Examples of items in the SDS are provided in Table 8-2. The learner completes the tool after participating in a simulation. The design features rated by the learners include objectives/information, student support, problem solving/complexity, fidelity, and guided reflection/debriefing. These features are postulated by Jeffries (2005) as integral to positive learning outcomes in a simulation. Content validity of the instrument was determined by a panel of nine nurse experts. Cronbach's alpha was computed to assess internal consistency and reliability for each scale. The coefficient alpha for the overall scale was 0.94.

Table 8-2 Sample Items from the Simulation Design Scale (SDS)						
Component	Sample Items	5	4	3	2	1
	SA - strongly agree A - Agree N - Neutral D - Disagree SD - Strongly Disagree	SA	A	N	D	SD
Objectives/Information	I clearly understood the purpose and objectives of the simulation.					
	The cues were appropriate and geared to promote my understanding.					
Student Support	My need for help was recognized.					
	I was supported in the learning process.					
Problem Solving/Complexity	I was encouraged to explore all possibilities during the simulation.					
	The simulation provided me with an opportunity to set goals for the patient.					
Fidelity	The scenario resembled a real-life situation.					
Guided Reflection/Debriefing	Feedback provided was constructive.					

Simulation Evaluation During the Implementation Phase

When simulations are implemented, particular components need to be included to ensure a good learning experience, student satisfaction, and good performance by the learners. According to Chickering and Gamson (1987), incorporating principles of best practice in education helps educators implement quality teaching activities and improve student learning. Educational practices are considered a very important component of the learning environment. To measure this component, the Educational Practices Simulation Scale (EPSS) was developed (see Table 8-3). The EPSS is a 16-item tool that the learner completes after a simulation. This tool measures the extent to which principles of best practice in education are being used in simulations; although, as a result of factor analysis, the original seven principles (Chickering & Gamson) have been collapsed into four factors.

The elements being evaluated in the EPSS scale are active learning, diverse ways of learning, high expectations, and collaboration. The questionnaire was tested for validity and reliability. The content validity was established through a review by nine nurse experts. The coefficient alpha, Cronbach's alpha, was 0.92. Table 8-4 provides sample items from the EPSS that reflect each of the four educational practices.

Table 8-3 Educational Practices in Simulation Scale (EPSS)		
Components	Description	Examples
Active Learning	Through simulation, learners are directly engaged in the activity and obtain immediate feedback and reinforcement of learning. Learning activities can range from simple to complex. Case scenarios, simulation of real-life clinical problems requiring assessment and decision-making skills, roleplaying with actors, and critiquing one's or a peer's videotape of a selected skill performance are examples of methods faculty can use to promote active learning (Cioffi, 2001; Lee & Lamp, 2003; Nehring, Lashley, & Ellis, 2002; Vandrey & Whitman, 2001). Such active and interactive learning environments encourage students to make connections between concepts and engage them in the learning process.	In a case scenario in which an intubated patient is restless, agitated, and coughing, affecting his oxygenation status, students can be asked to select the most appropriate intervention and describe the rationale for the intervention. The patient simulator can support more complex active learning strategies since the opportunity allows students to assess a critical health incident (e.g., collapsed lung or status asthmaticus) through the measurement of physiological parameters and communication with the "patient," on-the-spot planning for quick and appropriate nursing interventions, and real-time response by the simulator for realistic evaluation and further intervention (Nehring et al., 2002).
Diverse Ways of Learning	Simulations should be designed to accommodate diverse learning styles and teaching methods and allow students and groups with varying cultural backgrounds to benefit from the experience.	Design a scenario that has visual, auditory, and kinesthetic components. For example, use a monitor or lab reports (visual), program a patient simulator conversation about his symptoms (auditory), and require a procedure to be done (kinesthetic).
High Expectations	High teacher expectations are important for students during a learning experience because expecting students to do well becomes a self-fulfilling prophecy. Students should set goals with faculty and seek advice on how to achieve those goals. When both faculty and students have high expectations for the simulation process and the outcomes, positive results can be achieved.	Set up a scenario with multifaceted patient problems for the learner who needs to be challenged and needs to advance to the next level of knowledge and skills. Vandrey and Whitman (2001) assert that nurses can be pushed to expand their competency levels and empowered to achieve greater learning in a safe learning environment.
Collaboration	Collaboration is pairing students in a simulation to work together. Roles are assigned so that students jointly confirm assessments, make decisions about interventions, and evaluate outcomes.	An example of collaboration is assigning a student the role of primary nurse and a third-year medical student the role of primary physician. Place the two students in a setting where they will be confronted with a deteriorating patient for whom decisions need to be made, interventions need to be performed immediately, and assessments need to be done quickly and accurately.

Table 8-4 Sample Items from the Educational Practices in Simulation Scale (EPSS)						
Component	Sample Items	5	4	3	2	1
	SA - strongly agree A - Agree N - Neutral D - Disagree SD - Strongly Disagree	SA	A	N	D	SD
Active Learning	I actively participated in the debriefing session after the simulation.					
Diverse Ways	I received cues during the simulation in a timely manner.					
of Learning	The simulation offered a variety of ways in which to learn the material.					
High Expectations	The objectives for the simulation experience were clear and easy to understand.					
Collaboration	I had the chance to work with my peers during the simulation.					

The SDS and EPSS have been used extensively in practice and research. Schlairet (2011) completed an evaluation of the undergraduate curriculum utilizing the SDS and EPSS (Cronbach alpha 0.962 and 0.944, respectively). One hundred fifty baccalaureate nursing students in the traditional and accelerated program tracks participated in the evaluation. Through this evaluation, Schlairet identified the design characteristics that were most important to students and utilized this information to make modifications to the curriculum regarding simulation integrations. According to students in this study, active learning, high expectations, collaboration, and diverse learning were identified as important. Smith and Roehrs (2009) utilized the SDS in a descriptive correlational design study with 68 baccalaureate students in a traditional program. In this study, the students reported positive feelings about the five design characteristics with guided reflection having the highest mean score. Swenty and Eggleston (2011) conducted a study to determine students' perception of active learning and fidelity with simulation scenarios utilizing SDS and EPSS tools. Students indicated that active learning presence of realism (fidelity) were important.

Selected instrument to use during the implementation phase: Educational Practices Simulation Scale (EPSS)

Simulation Evaluation During the Outcomes Phase

While it is essential to evaluate the design and implementation of simulation activities, there is an acute need for effective evaluation strategies that focus on learning outcomes from simulation (Decker, Sportsman, Puetz, & Billings, 2008). Learning outcomes can be defined in a variety of ways, ranging from the learners' perceptions of the simulation activity to how the use of simulation as a teaching and learning strategy results in organizational-level functioning. Kirkpatrick (1994) referred to four levels of outcome evaluation, including (a) reaction, (b) learning, (c) behavior change, and (d) results.

Reaction: Learner satisfaction and self-confidence

Many educational researchers have been interested in learners' reactions to learning activities because when students are satisfied with their learning, their performance is higher (Chickering & Gamson, 1987). Student satisfaction with simulation activities can be evaluated using quantitative or qualitative measures of students' responses to the experience. Engum, Jeffries, and Fisher (2003); Jeffries, Woolf , and Linde (2003); and Johnson, Zerwic, and Theis (1999) all asked students to rate various aspects of an interactive computer experience on five- to six-point Likert scales. Overall, the studies showed that the students were very satisfied with this learning experience. Typical responses were that the experience provided opportunities to "think on your feet," "apply critical thinking skills," and "realize how much I really knew." In Cordeau's qualitative study (2010), the students viewed the simulation as an effective strategy to prepare them for practice, as evidenced by the following comments: "great help to my nursing career" and "found areas where I should improve to help my patients in real life" (p. 13). Similarly, qualitative results from junior and senior students using a human birthing simulator expressed satisfaction in open-ended questions. They reported that they enjoyed having "to work through steps" and "prioritizing" and that the experience seemed "real-life."

Educators have long been interested in how students react to simulation activities in terms of how they affect student self-confidence (Aronson, Rosa, Anfinson & Light, 1997 Cioffi, 2001; Johnson et al., 1999; Peterson & Bechtel, 2000; Thiele, Holloway, Murphy, Pardavis, & Stuckley, 1991). Researchers have found that placing students in simulated clinical situation allows the students to think critically and solve realistic problems. This practice, in turn, improves their self-confidence in these areas (Johnson et al.). An example of a study that evaluated the impact of a simulation versus a traditional learning activity in the promotion of self-confidence is Alfes (2011). In this study, students participating in the simulation were statistically more self-confident than the control group. Similar results were found by McCaughey and Traynor (2010) with 92 percent of the students reporting increased confidence in clinical judgment.

Learning: Introduction

One of the critical questions related to the use of simulation in nursing education is how it impacts learning. This area of outcome evaluation corresponds with Kirkpatrick's (1994) level two: learning. Educators and researchers measure learning outcomes from simulation activities using observation-based evaluations during simulation activities and questionnaires or other reflective assignments during or after simulation activities. To effectively evaluate learning outcomes from simulation activities, educators must clearly define what aspects of learning they seek to measure. These may include progress in the affective, cognitive, or psychomotor domains. Further, learning outcomes may include the development of specialized abilities such critical thinking, clinical judgment, communication, or teamwork.

It should be noted that while evaluation of learning in each of the domains (affective, cognitive, and psychomotor) is described separately, most observation-based simulation evaluation instruments focus on multiple domains. For example, to evaluate a student's ability to perform a skill (psychomotor), one will likely also be evaluating her knowledge (cognitive) about the procedures involved in the skill. Likewise, a thorough evaluation of students' overall learning will include multiple evaluation methods. An example from the literature of this can be found in Jeffries et al.'s (2011) research with advanced practice nurses where they assessed cognitive, affective, and psychomotor learning. The following will briefly describe each of the domains and abilities and examples of how one might measure learning in each.

Learning: Affective domain

Oermann and Gaberson (2006) described learning in the affective domain as "the development of values, attitudes, and beliefs consistent with standards of professional nursing practice" (p. 16). Affective learning overlaps with Kirkpatrick's level one, "reaction to the learning activity." Thus, the NLN Student Satisfaction and Self Confidence in Learning Scale (previously described) is one example of an instrument that may be used to evaluate learning in this domain. Further, Arnold et al. (2009) developed and implemented a 17-item Emergency Response Confidence Tool to assess students' confidence (from 0 percent to 100 percent) in their ability to perform specific tasks associated with emergency response scenarios. Data from this tool was then used to complement performance data collected using the authors' Emergency Response Performance Tool (Arnold et al.).

Many other authors have developed qualitative and quantitative instruments and questionnaires for measuring learners' perceptions of HPS learning experiences (Bambini, Washburn, & Perkins, 2009; Lambton, Pauly, O'Neill, & Dudham, 2008; McCausland, Curran, & Cataldi, 2004; Mole & McLafferty, 2004; Schoening, Sittner, & Todd, 2006). Additionally, Leigh (2008) published an entire literature review related to the effect of the human patient simulator HPS on students' self-efficacy, and Altshuler and Kachur (2001) reported on observation-based evaluations of how medical residents demonstrated cultural competency skills during objective structured clinical examinations (OSCE).

Evaluating learning outcomes in the cognitive domain can be highly subjective. Students' self-reports of satisfaction with learning activities may be motivated by the desire to provide socially acceptable answers to questions about their experience. Likewise, reports of self-confidence and self-efficacy may not correlate with competence. Theoretically, enhanced self-confidence and self-efficacy should correlate with superior performance (Bandura, 1989); however, simulation research is not conclusive in this area. The literature is still lacking in evidence about how confidence and behaviors associated with cultural competency and empathy demonstrated in simulation transfer to the clinical setting (Weaver, 2011).

Selected instruments for measuring learning in the affective domain: Student Satisfaction and Self Confidence in Learning Instruments and Arnold et al. (2009) Emergency Response Confidence Tool.

Learning: Cognitive domain

Learning in the cognitive domain includes both basic, factual learning, such as knowledge acquisition, and advanced learning, such as comprehension, application, synthesis, and evaluation (Jeffries & Norton, 2005). Bramble (1994) suggested that participation in simulations encourages higher-level thinking than the simple, low-level memorization of facts. To evaluate if the learner has achieved knowledge outcomes, faculty might use verbal questioning or concept/mind mapping (Billings & Halstead, 2005) to allow the learner to demonstrate understanding of concepts and explain the rationale for her or his actions. Another common strategy to evaluate knowledge is the written test which may be in the form of a pretest/post-test, post-test only, or pretest/post-test/one week post-test. According to Bloom's taxonomy (Yoder, 1993), multiple-choice knowledge exams can be written to assess different levels of knowledge attainment, including analysis, synthesis, and application. The higher the level, the more the student has to apply and synthesize the knowledge gained. Instruments designed to measure cognitive learning from HPS vary from unstructured questions, concept maps, and written knowledge exams to sophisticated measures of performance that incorporate cognitive learning.

Examples from the literature of instruments in the former categories include the use of faculty-designed activities and basic knowledge questionnaires listed in the questionnaires section of this chapter. Examples of instruments in the latter category include a variety of observation-based instruments. These instruments are commonly checklists that resemble OSCEs. Some examples of observation-based instruments from the literature that incorporate the evaluation of cognitive learning include Wolf et al.'s (2011) Simulation Faculty Grading Guidelines, Clark's (2006) Clinical Simulation Rubric© (Gantt, 2010) which is based on Benner's (1982, 1984) levels of nursing expertise, and Radhakrishnan, Roch, and Cunningham's (2007) Clinical Simulation Evaluation Tool (CSET), designed to measure clinical performance in the following areas: safety, prioritization, interventions, delegation, communication, and basic and problem-based assessment. One key to effective evaluation of cognitive learning using observation-based evaluation instruments is to ask students to verbalize the thinking behind their observable actions. This can take place during the simulation as "thinking out loud" or during the debriefing session when students provide rationale for their behaviors.

Regardless of the form of evaluation selected to measure cognitive learning outcomes, it is important to reflect on how the simulation is designed to contribute to or allow students to demonstrate learning in the cognitive domain. Simulation may be used as the teaching strategy, evaluation strategy, or both. If the educator is seeking a learning activity to help students memorize normal and abnormal lab values, less elaborate strategies than simulation may be warranted for both teaching and evaluation. However, if the goal is to allow students to demonstrate their ability to interpret a critical lab value and respond appropriately, simulation may provide an ideal opportunity for students to practice and educators to evaluate students' cognitive abilities.

Selected instruments for measuring learning in the cognitive domain: appropriate series of knowledge exam questions (e.g., HESI questions), performance-based instruments that incorporate the evaluation of cognitive learning such as Clark's (2006) Clinical Simulation Evaluation Rubric©.

Learning: Psychomotor domain

A simulation experience or laboratory is an ideal setting for students to develop and demonstrate psychomotor skills without risking harm to patients. Further, research indicates that simulation may lead to quicker acquisition of psychomotor skills than conventional training methods (Ost et al., 2001). Jeffries and Norton (2005) described psychomotor learning as including the development of technical skills that may incorporate affective and cognitive learning. Evaluation of psychomotor learning may include the use of checklists as measures of skill competencies (Jones, Cason, & Mancini, 2001) and may overlap with evaluation of learning in the cognitive domain because students must have knowledge to perform a skill or behavior.

Examples of instruments designed to measure learning in the psychomotor domain range from simple to complex, and cover everything from basic hand washing (Tollefson, 2010) to core outcome competencies in medical education (Rosen, Salas, Silvestri, Wu, & Lazzara, 2008). The latter instrument, the Simulation Module for Assessment of Residents Targeted Event Responses (SMARTER), is based on the Accreditation Council for Graduate Medical Education and was designed specifically for performance measurement in simulations. Additional examples of instruments designed to evaluate learning in the psychomotor domain include Murray et al.'s (2002) instrument to evaluate medical students' and residents' clinical performance in trauma simulations, Sevdalis et al.'s (2009) Imperial College Assessment of Technical Skills for Nurses (ICATS-N), and Liaw, Scherpbier, Klainin-Yobas, and Rethans's (2011) Rescuing A Patient In Deteriorating Situations (RAPIDS), an instrument designed to evaluate performance during a simulated clinical deterioration.

Other examples of instruments used to evaluate psychomotor skills that are routinely used in practice and research are the American Heart Association Basic Life Support (BLS) and Advanced Cardiac Life Support (ACLS) performance evaluation tools. Instruments designed to measure specific learning outcomes in the psychomotor domain are often adaptable for broader use. For example, an instrument used to evaluate medical students in a trauma simulation may be adapted to evaluate nursing students. However, as with all evaluation instruments, it is important to assess the validity and reliability of data under the specific set of circumstances that the instrument is proposed to be used.

Selected instruments to measure learning outcomes in the psychomotor domain: Clinical skills checklists and American Heart Association performance evaluation tools.

Learning: Critical thinking and related constructs

Some of the most common outcome measures described in the simulation literature are related to critical thinking. Although the specific outcome criteria vary from one study to the next, most have found that critical thinking does occur in the context of simulation activities (Bruce, Bridges, & Holcomb, 2003; Chau et al., 2001; Jenkins & Turick-Gibson, 1999; Johnson et al., 1999; Peterson & Bechtel, 2000; Rauen, 2001; Ravert, 2002; Weis & Guyton-Simmons, 1998). Many studies have used Facione and Facione's (1996) California Critical Thinking Skills Test (CCTST) (Chau et al.) or California Critical Thinking Disposition Inventory (CCTDI) (Ravert, 2008), or an instructor-developed critical thinking inventory and student journals (Jenkins & Turick-Gibson) to assess students' critical thinking abilities. Measuring critical thinking is of interest to nurse educators because it is an essential behavior in most nursing curricula.

Other concepts that parallel critical thinking and are being explored by nursing educator researchers include clinical judgment (Ironside & Jeffries, 2010), clinical diagnostic reasoning, clinical reasoning, and other concepts of higher order of thinking. Kuiper, Heinrich, Matthias, Graham, and Bell-Kotwell's (2008) Outcome Present State Model Debriefing tool is a computer-based worksheet designed to measure clinical reasoning and the Lasater Clinical Judgment Rubric (Lasater, 2007) is an example of an evaluation instrument designed to measure clinical judgment as described by Tanner (2006). Although well defined, constructs such as critical thinking and clinical judgment are challenging to measure, and instruments designed to reflect students' abilities in these areas must be carefully assessed for validity and reliability.

Educators and researchers may also be interested in using simulation to teach and evaluate constructs such as teamwork, management, and prioritization. Like critical thinking and the related concepts described above, before measuring performance in any of these areas, it is essential to clearly define what is being measured. Examples from the literature of instruments used to evaluate aspects of team performance include the Ottowa Crisis Resource Management Global Rating Scale (Kim, Neilipovitz, Cardinal, Chiu, & Clinch, 2006) and the Team Survey used by Millward and Jeffries (2001). As practice initiatives and research funding opportunities continue to highlight the importance of multi- and interdisciplinary work, it will be important to continue to develop these areas of simulation evaluation. Programs such as TeamSTEPPS® and other safety initiatives provide exemplars of simulations valuable role in these areas.

Selected instruments to measure critical thinking and related constructs: Observation-based instrument: Lasater Clinical Judgment Rubric, Questionnaires: California Critical Thinking Disposition Inventory (CCTDI) and the California Critical Thinking Skills Test (CCTST).

Behavior in the clinical environment as a result of the simulation activity

While it is essential to evaluate if and how students learn from simulation activities, it is equally important to evaluate whether behaviors associated with this learning are transferred into the clinical environment. Evaluation of behavior in the clinical environment as a result of simulation activities corresponds with Kirkpatrick's (1994)level three evaluation: behavior. Harper and Markham (2011) argue that evidence about the transferability of knowledge, skills, and abilities learned and practiced in simulation is essential to the future acceptance and development of simulation as a teaching and learning strategy. They cite a number of studies that document the transfer of specific skills (such as endotracheal intubation) from simulation to the clinical setting, but advise that evidence is inconclusive. Studies suggest that a strong majority of students and faculty (Abdo& Ravert, 2006; McCausland et al., 2004) believe that knowledge, skills, and attitudes learned and demonstrated in simulation transfer, or at least contribute, to improved performance in the real clinical setting. However, Feingold, Calaluce and Kallen (2004) found an incongruence between students' and faculties' responses when asked about skill transfer; 100 percent of faculty agreed that skills learned in the simulated clinical environment would transfer to the patient care setting but less than half of students agreed.

To effectively evaluate behavior in the clinical environment as a result of simulation activities, educators and researchers must evaluate students in both the simulated and actual patient care environments. These longitudinal evaluations may include a range of strategies for measuring learning and performance in the affective, cognitive, and psychomotor domains. While this level of evaluation may be impractical for the individual nurse educator, institutions investing resources in simulation facilities, equipment, and personnel would be well advised to seek outcome data about the effects of simulation teaching and learning on behavior in the clinical environment.

Results in practice that take place because of the activity

Finally, in addition to evaluating reaction, learning, and behavior change, Kirkpatrick (1994) suggests that it is important to evaluate results that take place in practice. In the case of simulation, these results could be changes at the unit, institution, or organization level. Examples include patient care and economic outcomes impacting length of stay or numbers of adverse events. Shinnick, Woo, and Mentes (2011) echo Kirkpatrick's emphasis of the importance of this level of evaluation in their statement that "nurse researchers need to ask the question, so what? to move HPS studies to the level of empirical research to determine whether HPS improves student knowledge, critical thinking and as a result, patient outcomes." (p. 71). This level of evaluation will require a substantial investment of time and energy, as well as the support and cooperation of multiple institutions. However, the basic building blocks of such research will include the systematic processes for evaluation described in this chapter.

Evaluation: Issues Related to Instrumentation

Evaluations, whether they focus on the design, implementation, or outcomes of simulation, frequently use standardized instruments for gathering data. This chapter has described a range of different instruments from questionnaires and observation-based evaluation tools to attitude scales, journals, and anecdotal notes. To ensure the highest quality evaluation, it is essential to select appropriate evaluation instruments. This can be done by following the systematic processes described in this chapter and first identifying and clearly defining the construct to be evaluated. From here, an evaluation instrument appropriate for measuring that construct may be selected or developed.

Once a potential evaluation instrument is selected, it is important to investigate what evidence exists about the reliability and validity of data produced using the instrument. Many of the instruments identified in this chapter have been used previously in practice or research, and there are growing bodies of evidence that will help guide their future use. If there is not adequate information about an instrument, or if the evaluation requires the development of a unique instrument, it is important to assess the validity and reliability of data produced using the instrument. The following sections will describe the importance of validity and reliability in simulation evaluation and suggest strategies for assessing the validity and reliability of data from performance-based simulation evaluation instruments.

Validity

Validity of evaluation data refers to the degree to which evidence and theory support the interpretation of the data (American Educational Research Association [AERA], American Psychological Association [APA], & National Council on Measurement in Education

[NCME], 1999, p. 9). Traditionally, terms such as face-, criterion-related, construct, and predictive validity have been used to describe the various facets of validity. However, in 1999, the AERA, APA, and NCME presented new standards for types of validity evidence. These include evidence based on the following: test content, response processes, internal structure, relations to other variables, and the consequences of testing. The table below is adapted from Goodwin's (2002) table describing the five types of validity evidence and includes possible strategies for validation of observation-based simulation evaluations.

Table 8-5 Types of Validity Evidence and Strategies for Validation of Observation-Based Simulation Evaluation Instruments

Type of validity evidence	Examples of strategies for validation of simulation evaluations
Evidence based on test content	Ask someone who is an expert in the area being evaluated to review the content of the evaluation instrument and report as to whether the content: 1. Logically represents the area being evaluated; 2. Is a relevant, adequate, and appropriate reflection of the area being assessed; 3. Unfairly biases any group of individuals being evaluated by over or under emphasizing certain components of the area being evaluated.
Evidence based on response processes	Ask those who are completing the evaluation instrument to report on how they arrived at their chosen responses. Look for systematic differences between different groups of individuals completing the evaluation instrument or being evaluated with it.
Evidence based on internal structure	Examine relationships between items on the instrument and how they conform or do not conform to the area being evaluated. For example, are items that are meant to evaluate a related construct highly correlated? One analytic strategy that may be used is factor analysis.
Evidence based on relations to other variables	Look for relationships between evaluation results and other data that is intended to reflect the same construct. For example, individuals' scores on a written critical thinking exam would be expected to be closely related to their scores on the critical thinking section of a performance-based simulation evaluation instrument (convergent) while individuals' written critical thinking scores would be expected to be less closely related to their scores on the technical skills section of the same performance-based simulation valuation instrument (discriminant). Compare individuals' scores from a simulation evaluation with their scores from a clinical evaluation.
Evidence based on the consequences of testing	Ask, 'are the intended benefits of the evaluation instrument being realized' and 'have any unintended consequences (good or bad) of the evaluation resulted?'

*adapted from Goodwin (2002) p.103

The purpose of validity assessment is to examine how well data from an evaluation reflects the constructs that the evaluator is trying to measure. Validity is specific to the context of the evaluation, so when selecting a simulation evaluation instrument, it is important to focus on the validity of the data produced using a measurement instrument rather than the instrument itself. An instrument cannot be deemed "valid" or "invalid" because validity depends upon how the instrument is used. For example, a checklist designed and validated to evaluate a nursing student's critical thinking ability may not produce valid data about an expert nurse's critical thinking ability. Likewise, this same instrument, designed to evaluate nursing students' critical thinking, is not likely to produce valid data about a nursing student's ability to perform a specific technical skill. Finally, validity evidence may be accumulated over a period of time and contribute to the ongoing refinement a specific evaluation strategy or instrument.

Reliability

Reliability is essentially a measure of consistency or the extent to which differences in individuals' scores produced using an evaluation instrument are consistent with differences in their true abilities (Furr & Bacharach, 2008, p. 82). One of the key strengths of using simulation for performance evaluation is the ability it affords educators to provide students with consistent opportunities to demonstrate clinical performance. However, this consistency must be accompanied by reliable evaluation methods to produce valuable evaluation data.

Observation-based evaluations are influenced by characteristics of both the individual being evaluated and the person completing the evaluation (Landy & Farr, 1980). Specifically, the reliability of data produced from observation-based performance evaluation instruments may be threatened by the impact of human perception. For example, one rater may perceive a student's performance differently than another rater, which may result in inconsistent or unreliable ratings between raters (Shrout & Fleiss, 1979). Likewise, an individual rater may perceive a similar performance or interpret an evaluation instrument differently on separate occasions, which may result in inconsistencies over time.

For these reasons, it is important to train raters and assess the reliability of data produced using observation-based evaluation instruments. The table below describes three types of reliability assessments and strategies for obtaining reliability evidence.

Table 8-6 Types of and Strategies for Obtaining Reliability Evidence	
Type of reliability evidence	Strategies for obtaining reliability evidence
Test retest (intra-rater) "If a measure truly reflects some meaningful construct, it should evaluate that construct compa-rably on separate occasions." (DeVellis, 2003, p. 43)	Ask individual raters to view and score a video-recorded simulation using an evaluation instrument on two separate occasions (separated by an adequate amount of time) and compare the ratings for consistency.
Inter-rater Properly training raters can increase inter-rater reliability. Raters must understand the construct they are tasked with evaluating and the evaluation instrument they are using.	Ask a group of raters to view and score the same simulation performance using the same evaluation instrument and compare ratings for consistency. Individual raters should not be allowed to interact when completing the evaluation.
Inter-instrument This form of reliability may be interpreted to reflect validity evidence based on relations to other variables.	Ask individual raters to view and score a simulation using two evaluation instruments that were designed to measure similar or different constructs. Compare ratings for convergent or discriminate validity.

Validity and reliability are highly inter-related. It should also be noted that data from an instrument can be reliable but not valid. This would be the case, for example, if a measuring tape consistently read that a penny was three inches thick. Like validity, the reliability of data is population specific. If an instrument has been assessed for reliability with one population of raters or individuals being rated, those results may not be generalizable to another population of raters or individuals being rated.

SUMMARY

Systematic evaluations of simulation design, implementation, and outcomes are imperative to the effective use and continued growth of simulation in nursing education. With the proliferation of simulation in nursing curricula, nurse educators and researchers must carefully evaluate how simulation contributes to the ultimate goal of nursing education — preparing nurses for practice. While simulation is currently used primarily for teaching and formative evaluations, nurse educators need to develop valid and reliable strategies for performance evaluation and make evidence-based decisions about the role these evaluations should play in every stage of the educational process— from beginning skills to end of program competency demonstrations and licensure. Will simulations become a required part of clinical teaching, learning, and licensure? Will simulations provide additional opportunities to extend learning in collaborative ways with other health care disciplines? Whatever the final consensus, there is a need to teach and effectively evaluate decision-making and problem solving skills that will lead to the continued growth of simulation in nursing education.

REFERENCES

Abdo, A., & Ravert, P. (2006). Student satisfaction with simulation experiences. *Clinical Simulation in Nursing, 2*(1).E13-316. doi:10.1016/j.ecns.2009.05.009

Alfes, C. M. (2011). Evaluating the use of simulation with beginning nursing students. *Journal of Nursing Education, 50*(2), 89-93.

Altshuler, L., & Kachur, E. (2001). A culture OSCE: Teaching residents to bridge different worlds. *Academic Medicine, 76*(5), 514.

American Educational Research Association, American Psychological Association, and National Council on Measurement in Education (1999). *Standards for educational and psychological testing.* Washington, DC: American Educational Research Association.

American Heart Association. (2011). BLS for healthcare providers. Dallas, Tex.: American Heart Association. In www.heart.org. Retrieved July 5, 2012 from http://www.heart.org / HEARTORG/CPRAndECC/HealthcareTraining /BasicLifeSupportBLS/BLS-for-Healthcare-Providers---Classroom_UCM_303484_Article.jsp.

Arnold, J. J., Johnson, L. M., Tucker, S. J., Malec, J. F., Henrickson, S. E., & Dunn, W. F. (2009). Evaluation tools in simulation learning: Performance and self-efficacy in emergency response. *Clinical Simulation in Nursing, 5*(10), e35-e43 doi:10.1016/j.ecns.2008.10.003

Aronson, B., Rosa, J., Anfinson, J., & Light, N. (1997). A simulated clinical problem-solving experience. *Nurse Educator, 22*(6), 17-19.

Bambini, D., Washburn, J., & Perkins, R. (2009). Outcomes of clinical simulation for novice nursing students: Communication, confidence, clinical judgment. *Nursing Education Perspectives, 30*(2), 79-82.

Bandura, A. (1989). Regulation of cognitive processes through perceived self-efficacy. *Developmental Psychology, 25*(5), 729e-735.

Barrows, H.S., & Feltovich, P.J. (1987). The Clinical Reasoning Process. *Medical Education 21*(2), 86-91.

Benner, P. (1982). From novice to expert the Dreyfus Model of Skill Acquisition. *American Journal of Nursing, 82*, 402-407.

Benner, P. (1984). *From novice to expert: Excellence and power in clinical nursing practice.* Addison Wesley Publishing, Plains: New York.

Billings, D. M., & Halstead, J. A. (Eds.). (2005). Teaching in nursing: A guide for faculty (2nd ed.). Philadelphia, PA: W. B. Saunders.

Bourke, M., & Ihrke, B. (2005). The evaluation process. In D. Billings & J. Halstead (Eds.). Teaching in nursing: A guide for faculty (2nd ed.) (pp. 443-464). Philadelphia, PA: W. B. Saunders.

Bramble, K. (1994). Nurse practitioner education: Enhancing performance through the use of the Objective Structured Clinical Assessment. Journal of Nursing Education, 33(2), 59-65.

Bruce, S., Bridges, E. J., & Holcomb, J. B. (2003). Preparing to respond: Joint Trauma Training Center and USAF Nursing Warskills Simulation Laboratory. Critical Care Nursing Clinics of North America, 15, 149-152.

Campbell, S. H. (2010). Clinical simulation. In K. B. Gaberson & M. H. Oermann (Eds.), Clinical teaching strategies in nursing (3rd ed.) (pp. 151-181). New York, NY: Springer Publishing.

Chau, J., Chang, A., Lee, I., Ip, W., Lee, D., & Wootton, Y. (2001). Effects of using videotaped vignettes on enhancing students' critical thinking ability in a baccalaureate nursing programme. Journal of Advanced Nursing, 36(1), 112-119.

Chickering, A. W., & Gamson, Z. F. (1987, March). Seven principles of good practice in undergraduate education. AAHE Bulletin, 39(7), 5-10.

Cioffi, J. (2001). Clinical simulations: Development and validation. Nurse Education Today, 21, 477-486.

Clark, M. (2006). Evaluating an obstetric trauma scenario. Clinical Simulation in Nursing, 2(2), e75-e77. doi:10.1016/j.ecns.2009.05.028

Courdeau, M. A. (2010). The lived experience of clinical simulation of novice nursing students. International Journal for Human Caring, 14(2), 9-15.

Davis, A. H., & Kimble, L. P. (2011). Human patient simulation evaluation rubrics for nursing education: Measuring the essentials of baccalaureate education for professional nursing practice. Journal of Nursing Education, 50(11), 605-611.

Decker, S., Sportsman, S., Puetz, L., & Billings, L. (2008). The evolution of simulation and its contribution to competency. Journal of Continuing Education in Nursing, 39(2), 74-80.

DeVillis, R.F. (2003). Scale development. Thousand Oaks, CA: Sage Publications.

Diekelmann, N. L., & Ironside, P. M. (2002). Developing a science of nursing education: Innovation with research. *Journal of Nursing Education, 41*(9), 379-380.

Engum, S., Jeffries, P. R., & Fisher, L. (2003). Intravenous catheter training system: Computer-based education versus traditional learning methods. *American Journal of Surgery, 186*(1), 67-74.

Facione N. C., & Facione, P. A. (1996). Assessment design issues for evaluating critical thinking in nursing. *Holistic Nursing Practice, 10*(3), 41-53.

Feingold, C. E., Calaluce, M., & Kallen, M. A. (2004). Computerized patient model and simulated clinical experiences: Evaluation with baccalaureate nursing students. *Journal of Nursing Education, 43*, 156-163.

Gaberson, K. B., & Oermann, M. H. (Eds.). (2010). *Clinical teaching strategies in nursing.* New York, NY: Springer.

Gantt, L. T. (2010). Using the Clark simulation evaluation rubric with associate degree and baccalaureate nursing students. *Nursing Education Perspectives, 31*, 101-105.

Goodwin, L. D. (2002). Changing conceptions of measurement validity: An update on the new standards. *Journal of Nursing Education, 41*(3), 100-106.

Hample, J., Herbold, N., Schneider, M., & Sheeley, A. (1999). Using standardized patients to train and evaluate dietetics students. *Journal of the American Dietetic Association, 99*(9), 1094-1097.

Howard, V. M., Ross, C., Mitchell, A. M., & Nelson, G. M. (2010). Human patient simulators and interactive case studies: A comparative analysis of learning outcomes and student perceptions. *CIN: Computers, Informatics, Nursing, 28*(1), 42-48.

Ironside, P. M., & Jeffries, P. R. (2010). Using multiple-patient simulation experiences to foster clinical judgment. *Journal of Nursing Regulation, 1*(2), 38-41.

Jeffries, P. R. & Norton, B. (2005). Selecting learning experiences to achieve curriculum outcomes, In D.M. Billings & J.A. Halstead (Eds.), *Teaching in nursing: A guide for faculty* (2nd ed., pp. 187-212). St. Louis, MO: Elsevier.

Jeffries, P., Childs, J., Decker, S., Horn, M., Hovancsek, M., Childress, R., . . . Politi, R. (2004, October). *How to design, implement, and evaluate simulations in nursing used as a teaching strategy.* Paper presented at the Education Summit, National League for Nursing, Orlando, FL.

Jeffries, P. R. (2005). A framework for designing, implementing, and evaluating simulations used as teaching strategies in nursing. Nursing Education Perspectives, 26(2), 28-35.

Jeffries, P.R. (2007). Simulations in Nursing Education: From Conceptualization to Evaluation, the National League for Nursing, New York: New York.

Jeffries, P. R., Beach, M., Decker, S. I., Dlugasch, L., Groom, J., Settles, J., & O'Donnell, J. M. (2011). Multi-center development and testing of a simulation-based cardiovascular assessment curriculum for advanced practice nurses. Nursing Education Perspectives, 32(5), 316-322.

Jeffries, P. R., Woolf, S., & Linde, B. (2003). Technology-based vs. traditional instruction: A comparison of two methods for teaching the skill of performing a 12-lead ECG. Nursing Education Perspectives, 24(2), 70-74.

Jenkins, P., & Turick-Gibson, T. (1999). An exercise in critical thinking using role playing. Nurse Educator, 24(6), 11-14.

Johnson, J. H., Zerwic, J. J., & Theis, S. L. (1999). Clinical simulation laboratory: An adjunct to clinical teaching. Nurse Educator, 24(5), 37-41.

Jones, T., Cason, C., & Mancini, M. (2002). Evaluating nurse competency: evidence of validity for a skills recredentialing program. Journal Of Professional Nursing, 18(1), 22-28.

Kardong-Edgren, S., Adamson, K., & Fitzgerald, C. (2010). A review of currently published evaluation instruments for human patient simulation. Clinical Simulation in Nursing, 6(1), e25-e35. doi:10.1016/jecns.2009.08.004

Kim, J., Neilipovitz, D., Cardinal, P., Chiu, M., & Clinch, J. (2006). A pilot study using high-fidelity simulation to formally evaluate performance in the resuscitation of critically ill patients: The University of Ottawa Critical Care Medicine, High-Fidelity Simulation, and Crisis Resource Management I Study. Critical Care Medicine, 34(8), 2167-2174.

Kirkpatrick, D. L. (1994). Evaluating training programs: The four levels. San Francisco, CA: Bernett-Koehler.

Klakovich, M. D., & Dela Cruz, F.A. (2006). Validating the interpersonal communication assessment scale. Journal of Professional Nursing, 22(1), 60-67.

Kogan, J. R., Holmboe, E. S., & Hauer, K. E. (2009). Tools for direct observation and assessment of clinical skills of medical trainees. Journal of the American Medical Association, 302(12), 1316-1326.

Kuiper, R. A., Heinrich, C., Matthias, A., Graham, M., & Bell-Kotwell, L. (2008). Debriefing with the OPT model of clinical reasoning during high fidelity patient simulation. International *Journal of Nursing Education Scholarship, 5*(1), Article 17. doi:10.2202/1548-923X.1466

Lambton, J., O'Neill, S. P., Dudum, T. (2008, October). Simulation as a strategy to teach clinical pediatricswithin a nursing curriculum. *Clinical Simulation in Nursing, 4*(3). doi:10.1016/j.ecns.2008.08.001

Landy, F. J., & Farr, J. L. (1980). Performance rating. *Psychological Bulletin, 87*(1), 72-107.

Lasater, K. (2007). Clinical judgment development: Using simulation to create an assessment rubric. *Journal of Nursing Education, 46*(11), 496-503.

Lee, C & Lamp, J. (2003). The use of humor and role-playing in reinforcing key concepts, *Nurse Educator, 28*(2), 61-62.

Leigh, G. T. (2008). High-fidelity patient simulation and nursing students' self-efficacy: A review of the literature. *International Journal of Nursing Education Scholarship, 5*(1), 1-17.

Lewis, D. Y., & Ciak, A. D. (2011). The impact of a simulation lab experience for nursing students. *Nursing Education Perspectives, 32*(4), 256-258.

Liaw, S. Y., Scherpbier, A., Klainin-Yobas, P., Rethans, J. (2011). Rescuing A Patient In Deteriorating Situations (RAPIDS): An evaluation tool for assessing simulation performance on clinical deterioration. *Resuscitation, 82*(11), 1434-1439.

Malec, J., Torsher, L., Dunn, W., Wiegman, D., Arnold, J., Brown, D. & Phatak, V. (2007). The Mayo high performance teamwork scale: Reliability and validity for evaluating key crew resource management skills. *Simulation in Healthcare, 2*(1), 4-10.

Marchigiano, G., Eduljee, N., & Harvey, K. (2011). Developing critical thinking skills from clinical assignments: A pilot study on nursing students' self-reported perceptions. *Journal of Nursing Management, 19*, 143-152.

McCaughey, C. S., & Traynor, M. K. (2010). The role of simulation in nurse education. *Nurse Education Today, 30*, 827-832.

McCausland, L. L., Curran, C. C., & Cataldi, P. (2004). Use of a human simulator for undergraduate nurse education. *International Journal of Nursing Education Scholarship, 1*(1), A23. doi:10.2202/1548923X.1035

Millward, L., & Jeffries, N. (2001). The team survey: A tool for health care team development. *Journal of Advanced Nursing, 35*(2), 276-287.

Mole, L., & McLafferty, I. (2004). Evaluating a simulated ward exercise for third year student nurses. *Nurse Education in Practice, 4*, 91-99. doi:10.1016/S1471-5953(03)00031-3

Morgan, P. J., & Cleave-Hogg, D. (2000). Evaluation of medical students' performance using the anesthesia simulator. *Medical Education, 34*, 42-45.

Murray, D., Boulet, J., Ziv, A., Woodhouse, J., Dras, J., & McAllister, J. (2002). An acute care skills evaluation for graduating medical students: A pilot study using clinical simulation. *Medical Education, 36*(9), 833-841.

Nehring, W., Lashley, F., and Ellis, W. (2002). Critical incident nursing management using human patient simulators. *Nursing Education Perspectives, 23*(3), 128-132.

Oermann, M. H., & Gaberson, K. B. (2006). *Evaluation and testing in nursing education* (2nd ed.). New York, NY: Springer.

Ost, D., DeRosiers, E., Britt, J., Fein, A., Lesser, M., & Mehta, A. (2001). Assessment bronchoscopy simulator. *American Journal of Respiratory and Critical Care Medicine, 164*, 2248-2255.

Peterson, M., & Bechtel, G. (2000). Combining the arts: An applied critical thinking approach in the skills laboratory. *Nursing Connections, 13*(2), 43-49.

Polit, D. F., & Hungler, B. P. (1995). *Nursing research: Principles and methods*. Philadelphia, PA: J. B. Lippincott.

Radhakrishnan, K., Roche, J., & Cunningham, H. (2007). Measuring clinical practice parameters with human patient simulation: A pilot study. *International Journal of Nursing Education Scholarship, 4*(1). Article 8.

Rauen, C. A. (2001). Using simulation to teach critical thinking skills: You can't just throw the book at them. *Critical Care Nursing Clinics of North America, 13*(1), 93-103.

Ravert, P. (2002). An integrative review of computer based simulation in the education process. *CIN: Computers, Informatics, Nursing, 20*(5), 203-208.

Ravert, P. (2008). Patient simulator sessions and critical thinking. *Journal of Nursing Education, 47*(12), 557-562.

Robertson, B. (2006). An obstetric simulation experience in an undergraduate nursing curriculum. *Nurse Educator, 31*(2), 74-78.

Rosen, M., Salas, E., Silvestri, S., Wu, T., & Lazzara, E. (2008). A measurement tool for simulation-based training in emergency medicine: The simulation module for assessment of resident targeted event responses (SMARTER) approach. *Simulation in Healthcare, 3*(3), 170-179. doi:10.1097/SIH.0b013e318173038d

Schlairet, M. C. (2011). Simulation in an undergraduate nursing curriculum: Implementation and impact evaluation. *Journal of Nursing Education, 50*(10), 561-568.

Schoening, A., Sittner, B., & Todd, M. (2006). Simulated clinical experience: Nursing students' perceptions and the educator's role. *Nurse Educator, 31*(6), 253-258.

Sevdalis, N., Undre, S., Henry, J., Sydney, E., Koutantji, M., Darzi, A., Vincent, C.A. (2009). Development, initial reliability and validity testing of an observational tool for assessing technical skills of operating room nurses. *International Journal of Nursing Studies, 46*, 1187–1193. doi:10.1016/j.ijnurstu.2009.03.002

Shinnick, M. A., Woo, M. A., & Mentes, J. C. (2011). Human patient simulation: State of the science in prelicensure nursing education. *Journal of Nursing Education, 50*(2), 65-72.

Shrout, P. E., & Fleiss, J. (1979). Intraclass correlations: Uses in assessing rater reliability. *Psychological Bulletin, 86*(2), 420-428.

Smith, S. J., & Roehrs, C. J. (2009). High-fidelty simulation: Factors correlated with nursing student satisfaction and self-confidence. *Nursing Education Perspectives, 30*(2), 74-78.

Swenty, C. F., & Eggleston, B. M. (2011). The evaluation of simulation in a baccalaureate nursing program. *Clinical Simulation in Nursing, 7*(5), e181-e187.

Tanner, C. A. (2006). Thinking like a nurse: A research-based model of clinical judgment in nursing. *Journal of Nursing Education, 45*(6), 204-211.

Thiele, J., Holloway, J., Murphy, D., Pardavis, J., & Stuckey, M. (1991). Perceived and actual decision making by novice baccalaureate students. *Western Journal of Nursing Research, 13*, 616-626.

Todd, M., Manz, J., Hawkins, K., Parsons, M., & Hercinger, M. (2008). The development of a quantitative evaluation tool for simulation in nursing education. *International Journal of Nursing Education Scholarship, 5*(1). Article 41.

Thomas M.D., O'Connor, F.W., Albert, M.L., Boutain D., Brandt, P.A. (2001). Case-based teaching and learning experiences. *Issues in Mental Health Nursing, 22*(5), 517–531.

Tollefson, J. (2010). *Clinical psychomotor skills: Assessment tools for nursing students* (4th ed.). South Melbourne, Victoria: Cengage Learning.

Vandrey, C. & Whitman, M. (2001). Simulator training for novice critical care nurses. *American Journal of Nursing, 101*(9), 24GG-24LL.

Weaver, A. (2011). High fidelity patient simulation in nursing education: An integrative review. *Nursing Education Perspectives, 32*(1), 37-40.

Weis, P., & Guyton-Simmons, J. (1998). A computer simulation for teaching critical thinking skills. *Nurse Educator, 23*(2), 30-33.

Weller, J. M. (2004). Simulation in undergraduate medical education: Bridging the gap between theory and practice. *Medical Education, 38*, 32-38.

Winters, J., Hauck, B., Riggs, J., Clawson, J., & Collins, J. (2003). Use of videotaping to assess competencies and course outcomes. *Journal of Nursing Education, 42*(10), 472-476.

Wolf, L., Dion, K., Lamoureaux, R., Kenny, C., Curnin, M., Hogan, M.A., . . . Cunningham, H. (2011). Using simulated clinical scenarios to evaluate student performance. *Nurse Educator, 36*(3), 128-134.

Yoder, M. E. (1993). Computer use and nursing research: Transfer of cognitive learning to a clinical skill: Linear versus interactive video. *Western Journal of Nursing Research, 15*, 115-117.

CHAPTER 9
SETTING UP A SIMULATION CENTER

Scott A. Engum, MD
Bruce Williams, RN, MS, MSN, EMT
Paul M. Collins, CCEMT-P

"The essence of education is not to stuff you with facts, but to help you discover your uniqueness, to teach you how to develop it, and then to show you how to give it away."

–Leo Buscaglia

INTRODUCTION

Modern simulation centers have become the centerpieces of teaching institutions. Accrediting bodies are continuing to increase support related to simulation and encourage innovative approaches in medical education. The simulation center, according to Infante (1985), is a replication of a clinical setting that allows the learner the opportunity to integrate theory and practice, think critically, and ensure patient safety. This learning environment is referred to by many names: skills lab, nursing lab, learning resource center (LRC), clinical proficiency center, learning center, simulation center, simulation lab, and clinical simulation lab. One primary role of the simulation center is to serve as a resource to faculty, professionals, and learners during development, implementation, and evaluation during simulation activities. This chapter will focus on the physical learning environment and the function of a simulation center, which includes collaboration, governance, organization, personnel, technology, space, supplies, resources, and equipment.

DEVELOPING A PARTNERSHIP

Partnerships involved in a simulation center come in all shapes and sizes in today's health care climate. It is uncommon for a single entity to "go it alone" in the development of a new center and may be very short-sighted in their mission or vision. A sole proprietorship simulation lab can limit simulation activities to one discipline and narrows equipment utilization, but could be the only option for some simulation users. There are multiple advantages in partnerships that relate to increasing revenue sources, improved opportunity for collaboration, opportunities for interprofessional activities, justification for specialized equipment (e.g. HarveyTM, vascular, and ultrasound simulators), and the ability to weave together the mission and vision of a health care system. This partnership can develop as a business type model such as for-profit, not-for-profit, governmental, or trust. An example of a simulation center partnership is the Simulation Center at Fairbanks Hall in Indianapolis where Indiana University Health, a not-for-profit facility, joined forces with Indiana University School of Nursing and Medicine. This incorporates over 1,000 nursing students, 1,000 residents, over 1,300 medical students, and hospital system professionals from three major institutions and numerous affiliates. This partnership contributed a total of $11.2 million for building and outfitting an interprofessional simulation center. The partnership encourages collaboration of administrators, educators, technicians, and end users to develop meaningful learning environments and valuable learning opportunities.

Challenges are present when combining multiple disciplines and can increase the complexity of a single shared mission, vision, goals, objectives, budget, established levels of accountability, scheduling priorities, and staffing responsibilities. None of these challenges should dissuade the pursuit of a relationship; however, the early acknowledgement of hurdles along the way will keep lines of communication open as the process proceeds.

FUNDING SOURCES

When beginning to think about the development of a simulation center, funding is a key issue. The budget and amount of funding available will dictate the size, the resources within the center, and the overall operations of the area. The initial funding for the simulation center construction and equipment can come from multiple sources and include items as reflected in Table 1.

Table 9-1 Examples of Funding Sources for Simulation Centers	
Funding Sources	Examples of the Sources
Philanthropic support	Professional organizations
	Industry
	Individuals
Grant funding	International
	Governmental
	Individual Foundation / Endowment
Institutional/Health Care System	School and/or medical center sponsorship
	Departmental grant
	Endowment
	Foundation grant
	Gift

The majority of funding will be spent on the building and equipping of the center. If the project can be incorporated into a current building initiative, money can be saved. Further revenue efficiencies can be realized if a center is able to take advantage of current purchasing agreements (hospital system) among the partners and industry. Maintaining a consistent, streamlined business and operational group can ensure steady progress within the project with minimal setbacks which ultimately may free up dollars for redistribution. Incorporating current business and development experts from a partnering system provides an efficient method to share in the project management and minimize hiring extra staff for the build-out and implementation phase. Lastly, utilizing available and relevant equipment within the system can free up capital to address the unexpected cost increase adjustments that are common in construction of a center.

ORGANIZATIONAL STRUCTURE

It is important to define the position of the simulation center in the hierarchy of the organization. This forethought will be important as health care systems grow, develop partnerships with affiliated providers, and begin discussions about multi-site simulation opportunities. Depending on a system and simulation center structure, it may involve various leaders from the organizations includes the deans of the individual schools, and high-level administration within a hospital system or board of directors. All though these individuals may be the primary support for the center, they likely report to executive leadership above them such as the vice president, president, or CEO of a hospital system or university. A clear understanding of who is ultimately responsible for the simulation center is important to gain buy-in, budgetary support, academic appointments, and to assist with personnel hiringand strategic planning of the organization's educational mission.

Day-to-day functions within a center will need to be maintained by the simulation center leadership committee and this often involves the director, coordinator or manager, educators, and information technology (IT) leadership. Frequent and regularly scheduled meetings are beneficial to discuss past, current, and future processes and concerns. An operational committee may also be of value to discuss more integral day-to-day issues that relate to work flow, assignments, schedules, simulation case concerns, and typically involves the manager or coordinator, technicians, IT support, administrative assistants, and schedulers. Having routine (weekly, bi-weekly), standing committee meetings allows for simulation center activities to be scheduled around these meetings to guarantee that all center individuals have input into process improvement. Below is an example of one hierarchy system:

- Executive Committee
- Governance Committee
- Leadership Committee
- Operational Committee

Open lines of communication from the executive level down through ancillary and operational services will keep the center operating smoothly. Regularly scheduled leadership meetings will be necessary to ensure the center is remaining on target with goals and objectives. Meeting with technicians and support staff on a recurring basis will promote a sense of belonging within the team. Frequent conversations at all levels will need to occur regarding work assignments, expectations, project deadlines, customer interactions, and active planning for future events, knowledge sharing, team building, and open dialog.

SIMULATION CENTER LOCATION

The allocation of space for a simulation center reflects the institution's commitment, need, and resources. Whether large or small, the simulation center space should accommodate multiple teaching and evaluation strategies that are selected based on the desired learning objectives and outcomes. The identification of potential teaching approaches will determine the exact needs of each simulation lab. The explosion of simulations in health care education is broadening and transforming the way these learning spaces are designed and equipped (Hyland & Hawkins, 2009; Kardong-Edgren & Oermmann, 2009).

With the teaching strategies identified, the design phase of simulation center development begins by assembling an interprofessional planning and design team. Depending on the environment, the team should consist of senior administration, facilities management, faculty, key educators, learner representative, simulation specialists, architect, technology consultant, audiovisual consultant, and business management personnel. The design team will need to keep several concerns in mind as they develop the plan for the new space.

Location of a simulation center is critical to ensure convenient use. Many institutions will have a broad set of users who are geographically separated, but share the same institutional Intranet system for similar needs and education. Options are to develop a single, centrally located center in the area of concentrated learners, or multiple key sites operating under a common administration. Each philosophy carries positives and negatives. If a multiple site model is chosen, this may afford lower scale renovations, customized equipment that fits that health care environment, and 24-hour access to the center by local users driving higher utilization. The cons associated to the multiple site model relates to the potential complexity for future accreditation because of the size and scope of center, duplication of services as well as equipment location, information technology and personnel, all adding cost to the system. If a single central site is chosen, this does allow for resources to be maximized and savings to be gained with efficiency of workforce and equipment; however, utilization by peripheral partners will be less as this mandates travel with its associated costs.

One of the first decisions is whether the space will be on site or off site. Each health care system will need to determine where their learners and customer base is coming from and determine the most efficient location for a new center. A second major issue relates to whether to renovate existing space or construct new space. Keep in mind that cost at times may be higher when attempting to renovate existing structures. The closer a system can place a simulation center to their customers and learners, the more ideal the ability to carry out educational opportunities as well as allow the learner flexibility to do independent activities. Maintaining a simulation center within the main teaching facilities limits transportation concerns for both learners and educators. However, it may also limit both parties from remaining fully immersed in the simulation center activity as they attempt to balance two worlds (real and simulated patient care). Being off site allows both parties to not feel torn between two necessities and remain focused in the simulation experience.

When a location is chosen, the group is often faced with the decision to build an independent structure or to combine with another project. These decisions are often made at a level above the design team; however, construction costs can be optimized if the parent organization incorporates the new simulation center space into an existing project as all construction entities are already on site. This does pose some concerns about logistics and maintaining timelines that may not be in the simulation center's best interest, however construction efficiencies can be maximized when potentially combined with another existing project. Secondly, if the combination project is incorporating educational space into their footprint, this may lessen some of the floor plan requirements the simulation center had initially scripted and will free up space for another purpose.

Renovation of existing space will always have limitations due to structural supports, ceiling height, established footprint and facilities infrastructure; however, each design team will need to work with the footprint allowed by the health care system.

FLOOR PLAN

Careful planning and preparation are necessary prior to commissioning the construction of a dedicated simulation center. It is important to plan for the best and worst case scenario 20 years into the future, as no one knows what changes will occur over time. Once the design and planning team has agreed upon the needs, location, and general plan, the architect will work with the team to develop a detailed space-by-space plan. It is critical for the design/planning team to visit multiple centers to view other floor plans, work flow as relates to the floor plan, and the educational space set-up. These trips will allow the design team the opportunity to talk about likes and dislikes of existing centers as well as allow all members to voice their concerns for the new center and design. These trips are invaluable for team building and will pay huge dividends later in the project when difficult decisions need to be made, and the center will have a high-functioning team because of this investment of time. This plan will include considerations as shown in Table 9-2.

Table 9-2 Considerations of Simulation Space Features
• Quantity and types of simulation space needed
• Who and how the space will be utilized
• Location in building and adjacent space of support areas (restrooms, elevator, freight)
• Support and other ancillary spaces (storage, office, IT)
• Equipment and infrastructure needed to support learning
• Special features (including door sizes, ceiling height, lights, tile, and more)

As centers are built, all design and planning teams must keep in mind future accreditation by governing bodies. One example relates to the American College of Surgeons (ACS) and the key components that must be met for accreditation as relates to space. Level 1 and 2 Institute requirements are briefly noted below. Level 1 criterion should be the space requirement goal when planning a facility, regardless if the actual ACS accreditation is desired.

Level 1 Comprehensive Education Institute (American College of Surgeons, 2012)

- Not less than 1,200 square feet dedicated space contiguous with a face to the public
- Not less than 4,000 square feet of additional space (conference rooms, storage, lounge, restrooms, lockers, kitchenette, and animate lab as needed)
- Space to accommodate a minimum of 20 trainees at a time with hands-on training
- Accommodate teleconferencing and teleproctoring
- Space to accommodate skills simulators
- Internet connectivity
- Administrative support staff space

Level 2 Basic Education Institute (American College of Surgeons, 2012)

- Is housed within a defined geographic location with all the components within proximity to one another
- No less than 800-1,000 square feet in size
- Space to accommodate a minimum of 6-10 trainees for hands-on training
- Identifiable space with access and signage for Education Institute

The actual space allocation will be determined by the anticipated use of learners and the community. Regardless of whether the space is located in an academic building, renovated hospital or clinical structure, several considerations are critical to enhance teaching and learning. The space should be column-free with good ventilation, flexible illumination, functional plumbing, and ample electrical support. The space should be easily accessible and have doors at least four feet wide. It should have external and internal corridors at least eight feet wide to allow for the movement of equipment.

The design of the space can be as basic as a bed and over-bed table, or as complex as a fully functional critical care unit with monitors, suction, and power columns. On average, a teaching unit should be no less than 85 square feet (a space that is large enough for up to four students to work together). Figure 9-1 provides a diagram of a typical teaching unit.

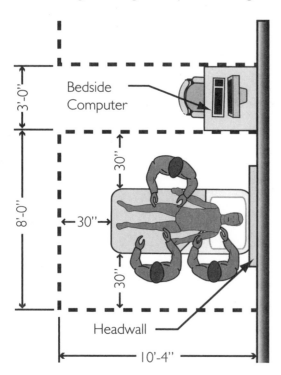

Figure 9-1
Diagram of Typical
Teaching Unit

The layout of the simulation center will depend on how the space will be used. An ideal space would be one that can take on a specific configuration for one teaching event, and then quickly transform into another setting to meet other teaching objectives. One concern that all design teams will need to consider is the location of specific types of simulation rooms and how to group them or position them within the center. One example is a pod configuration where four main areas of education have been intentionally structured so learners do not mingle during a simulation to limit inadvertent contamination of a scenario or training event (skills area, virtual clinic area, virtual hospital area, and acute care area). A thoughtful design (example shown in Figure 9-2) keeps learners in an assigned area therefore trying to maintain the fidelity of the simulation and minimize noise levels in the area. A second example of a pod configuration is an acute care area which houses the emergency room, intensive care unit, multi-purpose room, and operating suite with scrub room. Each of the acute care spaces includes a debrief room, support room, and simulation room (Seropian & Lavey, 2010).

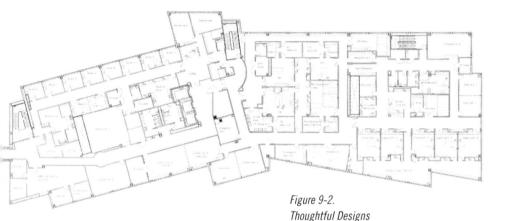

Figure 9-2.
Thoughtful Designs

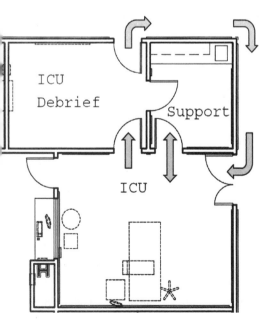

Figure 9-3 shows a common "pod" floor plan arrangement. This allows for pre-simulation discussion, simulation, and feedback/debriefing to occur in a circular loop affecting no other rooms around them. However, when desired, rooms such as emergency and intensive care can participate in joint education opportunities such as patient transfer and safe handoff with little effort from a floor plan perspective.

Figure 9-3
Common Pod Arrangement

Specialty spaces may be designed such as home care, perioperative nursing, maternal nursing, transport environments, or therapy areas. Other simulation spaces may be designed for multiple functions such as didactic learning and simulation space combined. If a space is to be used to perform physical assessments, the space will need to ensure privacy during practice sessions whether via privacy curtains, portable screens, or camera covers, and provide furniture for the patient or family member. Additional space modifications may be required to accommodate the needs of several teachers, larger learner groups, or diverse learner populations.

A separate control room area for carrying out and evaluating simulations is important. One issue a design team will need to consider is the number of control rooms within the floor plan. If each simulation space has a single control room, this will consume valuable real estate and limit the square footage available for simulation. Secondly, within the control room a simulation specialist will be needed to run the simulation therefore potentially increasing the need for specific resources to run the simulations as the number of control rooms may increase. Some centers develop a unified control room to cover multiple simulation spaces to optimize work flow efficiencies and save square footage for more important space designations. The control room usually has a one-way mirror into the simulation space that allows for a full view of the room by faculty, observers, and technicians. The lighting in the simulation space should consist of fluorescent lights over the bed and throughout the room. Consideration can be given to incandescent lights that can be dimmed remotely along with outlets to simulate a power outage. Natural lighting should be avoided in the simulation space because it can affect the quality of recorded events. In addition, natural lighting should be avoided inside the control room if using a one-way mirror. The control room will need to be darkened to prevent shadowed movements from being seen by the learners inside the simulation room. If natural light has been incorporated into these spaces, a high-quality blind or shade may be required to limit these effects.

Cameras should have wide-angle lenses and be wall- or ceiling-mounted with camera control (zoom and wide angle) from the control room. Cameras with a pan tilt zoom (PTZ) feature are recommended because of the flexibility and level of accuracy they provide during recording. When planning a room, simulation events may mandate relocating a camera in the space. This can be accomplished with ease in a tiled ceiling if ample cable length is left in the ceiling for each camera by the installers. A good rule of thumb is to leave the full length of the room in extra cable in the ceiling to permit physical camera repositioning to the opposite side of the room if necessary.

The recording equipment can be as simple as a VCR, DVR, security system, or a very complicated system with digital uptake feeds with sound mixer for audio quality. If using a complex audio visual system, all design planning must include adequate space for a technology room which includes server racks, additional electrical services, cooling and heating systems, cable trays, and an engineered floor to support the weight of the equipment. It is recommended that all simulation rooms have electrical outlets every four to six feet and include extra blank wall plates with wire chases installed before the walls are completed. Including these extra items upfront will save money and time as the center grows.

Developing a simulation center is a technologically driven venture. It is critical to have discussions with the architect, audio visual, software and information technology professionals about the needs for computer connections at work stations, in headwalls, control rooms, and many other locations around the simulation center. Limiting these discussions will require capital expenditures in the future and limit the growth of your center. Because microphones are most commonly ceiling mounted, it is essential to work with the architects to assure that the ventilation system for all rooms is quiet and that soundproofing techniques will be utilized for walls (carried higher into the ceiling and insulated to limit sound bleeding). One area that often escapes the design team is related to the location of pipes and vents within the ceiling. Discussing with the architect about all aspects of each room as relates to what is above the ceiling tiles is critical to minimize major water and sewer pipes as well as HVAC or air handler vents. These structures may be directly located where future mounting supports are required for operating room booms and weight lifting assistance devices. Moving pipes and vents in the future is costly when simple planning could avoid these errors during design.

A common area that is underestimated is the need for adequate storage space. When allocating space there are many strategic issues to keep in mind and the center needs to consider work flow, geographic activity areas, expected equipment sizes, and the need for alcoves. Additional items that need to be considered into storage allocation are beds, carts, intravenous poles, tables, crash carts, computer workstations on wheels, supply carts, linen storage, task trainer storage, wheel chairs, walkers, crutches, manikin storage racks, ultrasound machines, manikin tool area, and many others. Storage spaces should be well ventilated, well illuminated, have adequate electrical services, sink with running water and a reliable way to maintain security due to the unique nature of simulation equipment. Around the sink, it is common to have a prep space large enough to hold supplies, task trainers, and at times a manikin. For areas that are not in a secured room, such as cabinets in a patient room, lockable cabinets are beneficial. There will be multiple areas that have expensive IT and AV equipment that will need to be secured to prevent tampering and theft. Consideration should be given to efficient shelving units that are fixed and sturdy, in addition to mobile units that are extra wide (at least 24 inches deep) to assist in holding not only supplies, but also manikins, simulators, task trainers, and carrying cases. Designers and planners need to be aware that a portable cart will need to fit through doorways. So assure that the height of the door will permit cart pass-through prior to purchasing. In addition to storage, this area will likely be utilized for equipment maintenance, development, repair, and setup. A tabletop work space with direct lighting and extra electrical outlets adjacent to a deep sink is ideal, especially for cleaning and draining equipment due to the regular needs of flushing some equipment. Within the storage space, a portion of the room (ideally a central open area) can be utilized for manikin storage on a rolling cart. This allows for manikins to be racked for efficient storage and remain mobile due to the frequent need to move manikins from room to room. The weight of a manikin can be challenging for a single technician, and mobile carts assists with these transportation concerns. Whenever possible, place storage cabinets below windows and in challenged areas that have very little capability for simulation functions as this will allow the center to gain a tremendous amount of storage that was unanticipated.

Centralized areas of congregation (snack room or lounge), locker spaces, restrooms, and water fountains should be strategically spaced to minimize noise and control traffic patterns and congregation points. Noise is a critical factor that can be detrimental in maintaining fidelity and realism. Traffic patterns can add to the learner's experience or contribute to simulation contamination if learner groups mingle between simulation sessions.

HARDWARE AND SOFTWARE CONCERNS

Each center will be faced with the decision of what type of recording software to utilize to capture their simulation event. There are numerous vendors within the market and all offer a wide range of opportunities. First evaluate whether a system has the flexibility to support, maintain, and expand with a developing simulation center. There have been some successful centers with home grown audio/visual capturing systems. However, make sure there is proper support to keep a system running even in the event of personnel change, and that the cost required for setup and maintenance is in line with industry quotes. Often, custom made systems appear to be a cost effective approach, but the long-term functionality of these systems rarely keeps up with advancing technology. It is recommended that simulation centers interview each group, have them develop a business plan, and demonstrate their product. Following an adequate vetting by your design group, one particular product should have a better fit for your center based on functionality, ease of use, price, technology requirements, support needs, warranties, or long-term relationship. Every center has its own unique needs, so there is no one-stop shopping for this integral component. Table 9-3 provides examples of areas to think about.

Table 9-3 Hardware and Software Concerns	
Cost	Warranties
Support staff	Customer service availability
Maintenance	Hardware
Software	Product education
Software features	Equipment requirements
Company reputation	Advances in the field
Downtime of product and guarantees	What you can do locally
What requires the main company to service	What IT support is required locally

Along with the challenging decision of your audio/visual (AV) capturing system, the simulation center will need to partner with a hardware company to install all the needed equipment for simulation AV capturing. It is not uncommon for a software company to have a list of preferred vendors that they work with and that understand their product on a deeper level. However, a simulation center can choose who they feel fits their role and are not forced to participate with an associated vendor unless they desire. This hardware vendor decision can be just as critical as the software vendor choice.

The AV hardware company should methodically lay out a schematic footprint that the center will live with for years to come. The schematic should be challenged for long-term use and stability and functionality. Sometimes the most inexpensive plan on day one can be more costly in the future and could have significant limitations in functionality. Again, a design group should interview each vendor and compare "apples to apples." Ensure all vendors bring their products to the level you desire. This will allow the group to determine differences and cost break points and compare functionality. Once a vendor is chosen, the center will live with these individuals on a daily basis, so it is critical that there is a respectful working relationship.

Both the software and hardware companies will offer warranties for their services. It is advisable that new simulation centers obtain and maintain full functionality warranties until they have had adequate time within the system to determine the need and then to develop onsite support staff if it is chosen to not carry a warranty in the future. These systems are quite complex and it is typically advisable to maintain these warranties to keep full functionality 24 hours a day, seven days a week. It is critical to have these vendors servicing your facility not only regularly with routine maintenance, but when a system failure does occur during high stakes events. Prompt repair and problem mitigation should be expected. Failure to have warranties in place often places the simulation center at the bottom of the service list and usually results in higher costs and long delays for your customer base.

Personnel

Following the center's opening, a successful and thriving organization will need to integrate all personnel into the center's mission and vision. It is important to incorporate not only the educational, but also the clinical and research missions of the entity or partners into the simulation center fabric as many initiatives occurring within the simulation center will directly impact these initiatives. As health care systems are held responsible for improving patient safety and clinical outcomes, these items will undoubtedly be tied to simulation center educational initiatives to bring about improved communication and safer bedside care. The goal is to translate learning from the simulation center to the point of care, and the center's staff plays a vital role in that learning.

Staffing the simulation center is critical to the success of any operation. Depending upon a simulation center's size, organizational structure, and technological capabilities, staffing can be quite variable; however, this aspect of simulation center management can be your Achilles heel. Most centers function with a director who is typically part-time and not uncommonly a practicing health care professional (physician) who also has other responsibilities outside the simulation center such as a faculty position in an academic system. In addition, the director understands the curriculum and how the simulation center can help faculty meet their curricular goals and in many cases this individual is a member of the health care system or school's curriculum committee. The director can also serve on other appropriate committees that assist in advancing education as she or he will be able to assist educators with integrating simulation into a curriculum. It is common to see 50 percent of the director's time devoted to the administrative functions of the simulation center. In addition, it is critical to have a full-time manager or coordinator who is designated to manage the day-to-day operations of the simulation center. This individual must not only have the administrative skill set to manage employees and provide mentoring and coaching, but must also possess an advanced working knowledge of medicine, simulation planning, programming, education, debriefing, equipment function, and information technology framework.

Personnel requirements and qualifications will vary by facility. Simulation technicians, coordinators, and faculty will make up the core of your team. Job descriptions for each will simplify both hiring and the management of personnel. The simulation technicians will assist in all aspects of simulation scenarios. Technicians will need some key skills, such as the ability to understand medical terminology, interact with and program technology, interpersonal skills, computer skills, prioritizing and organizational skills. Technicians from many backgrounds, such as an emergency medical technican (EMT), paramedic, nursing, or out of college with degrees in media/audio/video or even engineering are hired in the technician position. The technicians must possess the skills to flexibly perform all tasks that evolve throughout the day and needed to operate a simulation center.

A center that follows a single-site model will need several technicians and a coordinator to assist with handling the larger volume of customers. Centers that function on a multi-site model can often operate with a director and fewer technicians who often recruit educators for assistance when there are larger events. The number of technicians relates to the number of events a facility wants to orchestrate. For a single high-fidelity room, the minimum number of support individuals is typically an educator and a simulation technician. Thus, the example of an emergency room interprofessional event running three rooms simultaneously would require three technicians and three educators. In a similar event involving an interprofessional virtual hospital ward with medical and nursing students, five rooms are running simultaneously and would necessitate 10 individuals involved. This is a major resource requirement for any simulation center and careful planning is necessary as any other activities in the center must be self-sufficient and need minimal technician support to happen simultaneously. Therefore, even in a center of 30,000 square feet, the coordination of high-fidelity technician needs in addition to running lower-level task trainer events allows for simultaneous simulation encounters to occur with high customer satisfaction and center staff working effectively and efficiently.

A multi-site system will typically pull all educators, the simulation center director, and the coordinator into the picture for large-scale events, to support overextended technicians. When not running a simulation session, a coordinator would assist with course coordination, as well as facilitating all other events, along with scheduling and public relations.

The majority of faculty for a simulation center will come from the clinical units, divisions, departments, or schools that utilize the center for training. Typically, the faculty are employed or appointed from their home institution and their salary and benefits are already addressed. The vast majority of faculty will be fulfilling their teaching mission and requirements for promotion and tenure and will be the driving force for new initiatives. It is common that these new users will need education about the simulation process, how to develop quality scenarios, equipment selection, manikin selection, the use of manikins, the process of how to run a scenario, and debriefing techniques. When instructed and mentored properly, these individuals will be the future champions in the simulation process.

All centers will need to determine their core workforce, which may include a mix of volunteers, full-time, part-time and supplemental employees. Full-time employees carry a 40-hour work week and full benefits package which can be anywhere from 25 to 40 percent of the salary costs depending upon the environment. Providing a comprehensive orientation program will require less supplemental training for each event, allow them to gain experience, confidence and become a loyal and dependable staff member who supports the mission, vision, and goals of the center. Employment costs should be built into the annual budget with a supporting job description. Careful tracking of center statistics will help to justify adding or releasing full-time staff. As center usage volumes change, these statistics can be invaluable when trying to justify additional staff, especially if there is a hiring freeze in effect. With economic downturns and health care budgetary cuts, it has become increasingly difficult to get permission from oversight committees for the addition of new staff.

When considering full-time, part-time and supplemental staff, a few items are important to keep in mind. Part-time employees typically work 20 hours per week, have partial benefits and after experience is gained, can be very valuable during flex times, as many of them have flexible hours and can adjust to center volume changes. A significant downside to part-time and supplemental employees is that each event will require planning, physical setup, implementation, and teardown. Many of these functions occur around other scheduled events, and sometimes a day or two ahead of the scheduled event which can put an additional workload on full-time technicians if the part-time technician does not have flexible hours. Some centers utilize active supplemental employees. These individuals work on an as-needed basis and are not eligible for benefits. If the simulation center is fully staffed with technicians, supplemental employees can be invaluable, filling in during high service times; they also lessen the financial burden because they do not carry benefit packages. However, a center should not rely on this type of individual as the backbone of services rendered.

There are times within all organizations when a specific type of expertise is required that may not be available within the simulation team and a contracted employee may be needed to fill this requirement. Information technology is one of those specialty areas in which the search for the proper individual may take time, but the services these individuals are responsible for are needed today. A simulation center can contract with an outside company to provide temporary expertise and the contracting company will carry all the benefits and employer requirements. One needs to understand that this method of coverage does come at a premium and may cost the simulation system 40 to 50 percent more. However, within the right area, this may be an excellent short-term solution until a long-term solution is determined or someone is trained.

If a simulation center is going to provide Objective Structured Clinical Examination (OSCE) with standardized patients who portray the role of human patients, then the vital role of standardized patient educator or coordinator needs to be established. This individual spends a significant amount of time working with customers who utilize standardized patients to plan the events, create proper scripts, evaluate checklists, and train the standardized patient for consistent role performance. Depending on the volume of learner encounters your system projects, this will likely be a full-time position.

Further staffing of the simulation center can take many forms and some individuals may have multiple duties depending upon resources, funding sources, center size, and capabilities. As simulation centers become busier, it is not uncommon for a receptionist to be required to direct educators and learners where they are scheduled, greet guests, and welcome tour groups. The receptionist can also assist in administrative functions to optimize efficiency.

Larger simulation centers may have business development and project management oversight support staff within the center. This revenue-producing position is a valuable asset for systems to use with strategic planning and budgetary oversight. If a center is unable to afford or maintain this type of person on the payroll, investigate utilizing the schools or hospital system's business department. Asking the business department for a specific person to be designated to the simulation center will allow for a relationship to be established. There are few simulation center business models available for review, so a resource person with business expertise can assist in developing appropriate guidance in this maturing area.

Volunteers are a valuable resource for all centers, large and small. These can be individuals who come from the community or even undergraduate or graduate students. All of these individuals provide valuable man hours to assist in carrying out the mission of the simulation center. It is not uncommon to have a graduate or undergraduate student develop innovative curriculum plans while doing volunteer or elective rotation work. In addition, college and high school students can assist simulation technicians in set up, implementation, and tear down after education.

Research assistance can come from many locations. If you are in an academic environment, each of the academic divisions typically has research personnel who can assist in carrying out projects. However, their simulation knowledge may be limited and selecting an individual with an education background may be beneficial. An educator may also have a research background that can be utilized to initiate new opportunities. If a primary researcher is funded, this could be part-time or full-time depending on the funding source. In either situation, the simulation center could fund the initiative under a global budget or share the cost with other educational systems to keep the center's budgetary funds intact.

Administrative support is necessary for recording keeping, ordering, invoicing, and employee timekeeping. This position's skill set will also depend on the center's size, capabilities, and organizational partners. A moderately busy simulation center of 30,000 square feet is capable of keeping an administrative assistant engaged with full-time assignments.

Very often dismissed are individuals who support the physical plant such as maintenance, janitorial, and facilities. Simulation activities cannot occur without proper support from all of these entities and often these expenses can be shared with other occupants of a building or campus. However, if a center is freestanding, these services will need to be included in the personnel hiring, budgeting, and management plan. One major decision will be whether these are employees of the center or contracted labor, and each center will need to determine their threshold for these services.

One critical concern relates to protected time for all simulation center employees and liaisons to carry out their functions. If an employee is full or part-time and simulation center based, their functions will be focused on center objectives. Managers and educators may have dual roles that mandate job sharing with dedicated time between multiple department and health care system environments. The success of a center will be determined by these individuals having adequate protected time to advance the causes of the simulation center. These times will need to be negotiated with their primary department.

OPERATIONS

Development of interprofessional relationships and activities within the simulation center depend on thoughtful, meaningful simulation leaders to promote interprofessional simulation activities and hiring the right personnel who understand the importance of developing, building, and maintaining these working relationships. A simulation center must operate with intention, finding ways to bring educators with varies backgrounds together. An example of this is to develop simulation center liaisons who are assigned by their primary employer (schools of nursing, medicine, and health care systems) to spend 50 percent of their time within the simulation center to develop, plan, create, implement, and orchestrate simulation education. By having these individuals in the simulation center, leadership meetings are able to focus on best practices from multiple disciplines, sharing ideas for curricular advancement, incorporating interprofessional simulation opportunities and simulation center advanced planning. These liaisons are critical contributors that must be identified in any center.

The technician staffing of the center for simulation events and training sessions can be handled in different ways. Within the training, there are numerous functions that need to be considered from taking a reservation from a preliminary request, running the event, and processing all the way through to completion. Producing a quality, structured event begins with a well-organized plan. Table 9-4 provides recommended steps for planning a simulation event.

Table 9-4 Steps for Planning a Simulation Event
1. Contact the customer and discuss new reservation
2. Provide a simulation template to the customer for development
3. Establish and confirm room needs, required equipment, and supplies
4. Determine adequate staffing for event
5. Review the submitted simulation template for completeness and clarify questions
6. Program any new software simulation needs
7. Support the educator as they develop support materials for the event
8. Establish a time table for the event day
9. Prepare set-up and tear-down notes
10. Address information technology requirements
11. Finalize with the customer any invoicing requirements

In most centers, the simulation technician is responsible for closing out an event, as this involves determining all billable items used that must be included on an invoice (e.g., hours of use, supplies, and hours of personnel), establishing the number of educators and learners who participated in the environment, and debriefing with the customer to assess areas of improvement for future events. This allows for a complete closure of the loop of services from initial request to final invoice.

Three environments exist within large simulation centers, including an outpatient center/ OSCE area that may require only one simulation technician to manage the information technology AV recording system, as this software is typically all-inclusive and more independent in function when compared to single simulation rooms. The second area is the high-fidelity simulation suite, where typically a single technician is required to manage operations to allow an educator to stay focused on evaluating learner performance and not the logistics of the event. Lastly, there are skills areas within most centers that can often run without the direct support of a technician outside of set up and tear down time. The number of simulation technicians, not the number of rooms, will be the limiting factor to the number of events you can carry out simultaneously.

Many new simulation centers underestimate the need for information technology positions in an effort to utilize the existing IT department of the school or hospital system. Initially this may seem to be an effective method to keep personnel budgets lower. However, the large amount of AV equipment and the large number of computer workstations in this type of environment frequently need specialized attention. In a 30,000-square-foot center, it is not uncommon to have over 130 computer workstations with different imaging and requirements, in addition to software and hardware failures. In addition, an in-house IT support person should interface with multiple servers, the recording software vendor, and communicate with the IT support companies. This specialized technology will need constant adjustments to keep it operating at peak performance. This is especially important when many vendors are off site and typically across the country. The high level of aggravation and man hours involved for someone to troubleshoot numerous problems is often not worth the cost savings of doing without an IT individual.

It is important to develop standard operating procedures for day-to-day operations, as well as addressing advertising and publicity and disseminating information. Continuous analysis of the operations, process, and outcomes will be very important for maintaining proper direction.

Transportation and parking are big factors for any center even when located on the main campus of a health care system. These concerns may not be the primary responsibility of the simulation center; however, all curricular activities will be affected by inefficiencies in these areas. If learners and educators are not able to efficiently find parking and get to the simulation center in a timely manner, these factors will always limit the center's ability to meet the needs of each learner group. Parking should be on site and adequate for all employees and participants. It is preferable to not be metered or pay for parking. Centers that are off campus will need to determine the method of transporting participants. This can be by a shuttle system (bus or monorail). However, adequate time for the participants to transition from one educational opportunity to the next must be anticipated and planned for. Secondly, if one of the transportation systems becomes inoperable due to weather or maintenance, an alternative needs to be in place for a smooth transition to maintain curricular progress.

Budgetary

Rigorous attention to cost containment and new revenue streams will assist in keeping the simulation center within budget. The simulation center administration will be responsible for developing the business plan and budget, and will provide a systematic process of review to ensure adherence. All centers will need to maintain consistent records and transparent communication with schools and hospital administrative leadership that are responsible for center oversight. When assessing the need for spending, always consider if the expenditure will support the educational mission, goals, and objectives of the center without creating an imbalance. Some centers find additional funding sources by attracting external partners and customers who will pay fair market value to utilize available spaces. These external relationships generate revenue to expand the center.

Revenue streams can come from multiple sources including inside and outside customer service agreements, research and educational grants, and donations from individuals, vendors, foundations, and others, to name a few. Most centers follow a collective business model where the organization is composed of a relatively large number of professionals in the same or related fields of endeavor, which pools resources, shares information, and provides benefits for their members. However, the "fee in, free out" business model has also been employed. In some systems, each partner pays a percentage of the annual operating budget up front. In this type of situation, all services are provided to that partner at no cost to the educator or learner groups, as all expenses are a fixed cost within the system. This takes tremendous pressure off the simulation center staff and educators to carry out curricular objectives and does not ration center usage for budgetary reasons.

Other centers might adopt a model that requires the center to be self-sustaining and all customers are invoiced for services. With a self-sustaining model, the majority of program decisions may be determined based upon budget and revenue sources. Tensions can mount in the fee-for-service environment, depending on the customer base, and advances need to be carefully and strategically planned, which may in some cases delay implementation, especially if awaiting customer budgetary approvals. Some have utilized a hybrid model where partners pay an annual fee, affiliate facilities pay a percentage of their use costs or a fixed per-learner use fee, and external, non-affiliated customers pay full service expenses at fair market value.

Lastly, grants and donations can be invaluable to a center as these can subsidize a systems budget. Grants and donations are not a guaranteed source of revenue and cannot be the cornerstone to build your center around. Long-term, strategic development is the foundation to ensure a simulation center's viability and sustainability.

There are major budgetary concerns that develop as a center matures and educators expand the curriculum. This is not a tremendous problem in a center where the costs are covered by the system; however, consumable expenditures can challenge a system. Below is a list of items that can challenge a budget if funding sources for these items are not planned for in advance. Usage and associated costs of these items have many variables, including but not limited to faculty orientation to the equipment, student volume, frequency of use, and conditions of use. For a list of additional budgetary considerations see Table 9-5.

Table 9-5 Simulation Lab Operations Budgetary Considerations
1. Standardized patients (cost approximately $16.15/hour)
2. Specialized equipment needs
3. New equipment warranties
4. Transitioned (donated to center) equipment warranties
5. In-situ simulation support by simulation center staff
6. Disposable supplies
7. Service life of equipment
8. Software and hardware advances
9. Server storage space
10. Inflationary expenses
11. Economic downturn or recession
12. Hiring freeze or budgetary cuts

CAPITAL EXPENDITURES

Capital expenditures are often mentioned at the time of opening a new simulation center. However, after all the excitement and glamour of opening a new center are gone, leadership soon realizes that an operational budget does not afford a center the ability to purchase capital expenditures. After a few years when equipment starts to wear and break down, new equipment will be required and a capital expenditure account will be necessary. The creation of a capital expenditure account should be discussed at the time the simulation center opens. This could be a yearly amount (use it or lose it) or a fund that remains intact with decreasing balance. Every center will need to negotiate the best opportunity available.

COST AND BILLING STRUCTURE

Unfortunately, the best business model for a simulation center has not been discovered and often, what will work in one environment will not work in another. Establishing a cost value for every function and service a simulation center offers carries a few benefits. First, it establishes a starting point as to what something costs and how much a customer will be charged to utilize a center. Profit can be built into any calculation in an effort to have future funds to advance education, increase personnel, and repair or replace equipment. If the cost structure is not utilized for billing a customer, then this data can be utilized to show return on investment for the services offered within the simulation center. Too often an administration leadership will ask how the simulation center is benefiting the health care environment and is the system getting its monies worth. It is difficult to trace single simulation events directly back to the patient bedside and a specific outcome, but the cost can be shown, and education services provided in relation to the budget that was expended to make that occur. In most centers, it would be expected that this is a net positive for services render.

EQUIPMENT

Careful selection of durable, recyclable, and disposable equipment will enhance the ability to simulate real clinical situations. All equipment selected should be in good operating condition and reflect current technology. The use of out-of-date and unfamiliar equipment makes it difficult for the learner to transfer skills and knowledge to patient care settings. For example, the use of an old patient-controlled analgesia (PCA) pump, which is no longer manufactured or used in the hospital, would not be appropriate for simulation use even if one could find the proper tubing and parts to service the unit. However, out of date equipment can be beneficial if the item continues to teach the principal objective of the educator.

When purchasing equipment, start with previously established relationships and consider trade-ins, teaching models, and using the purchasing power of a connected institution(s). Many pieces of equipment, when utilized for teaching, do not need to be certified for direct patient care. Often the company will sell that piece of equipment at a reduced rate and it will be labeled "not for patient use" to cover liability concerns, as the clinical engineering responsibilities lessen in such cases. Consider taking advantage of a local hospital systems' purchasing agreements with specific companies and the simulation center can negotiate and likely receive a more competitive purchase price. This can also be useful when the hospital system is either upgrading or sending in a new equipment order. In the case of an equipment model change, for example new defibrillators are chosen for the hospital system, all existing center defibrillators could be exchanged at no cost to the simulation center for the new and current model desired in the hospital. Another example is if there is a purchase occurring in regards to intravenous pumps, negotiations can occur where a specific number of units are assigned to the simulation center with reduced purchasing costs compared to buying solely for the simulation center. When selecting the durable medical equipment to be purchased, depending on your simulation center alignment (hospital, school, other), start by contacting a local purchasing representative for the larger entity to inquire about a list of vendors with approved relationships and pricing. This can expedite the process tremendously, and in some cases, price negotiations and ordering can be accomplished by the purchasing department. The following should be considered when selecting equipment:

- Who will be using the equipment and how often?

- Is the equipment used by a large number of clinical services?

- Are disposable materials necessary to the related equipment (e.g., tubing) and can it be purchased at a reduced cost?

- Are educational materials available for the equipment, or are there on-site, in-service classes so learners and faculty can learn to use the equipment?

- Is the company interested in donating, upgrading, or parking a usable loaner in the simulation center?

All of the equipment, if clinically relevant, will have sophisticated technology and the purchase and maintenance of the equipment can be expensive and labor intensive. Because of the limited funds that are typically present in simulation centers and limited technology resource individuals, one may want to consider renting, leasing, borrowing, or sharing equipment as a viable option to ensure access to specialized equipment when needed. One strategic maneuver to consider if the center is associated with a hospital system is clinical engineering. This department within the hospital is responsible for maintaining, repairing, and troubleshooting equipment and can lessen the load for simulation center personnel. In addition, this is budgeted by the hospital system and carries limited financial responsibility for the center proper.

DURABLE EQUIPMENT

Selecting state-of-the-art, durable equipment for purchase can be similar to buying a car. The same basic product is available from many vendors, and there is great benefit to "shopping around." Before purchasing equipment, it is essential to assess the equipment currently in use by local health care agencies and established programs on your campus that are likely to utilize your facility. One can look at the current equipment in these health care agencies to observe the interest in use, quality, and function in the real clinical setting and potential uses in the center. It is important to discuss purchases with the purchasing department to gain information, get the manufacturer's or distributor's name and contact information, cost of product, any special contractual agreement (e.g., tubing) related to the product, determine the reliability of the company with delivery, service, local representatives, and warranties, and lastly, determine the warranties available, and cost structure. Gaining all of this information will allow you to do "comparison shopping." When dealing with these vendors, it is important to alert them to where the equipment will be used, who the learners are, and to discuss their ability to offer a reduced price, donation, or some type of creative purchasing agreement (e.g., multiple item purchase and graduated reduction in cost). After review of all available information, follow your institution's policies related to procurement of durable equipment. One must keep track of the purchasing requests until the equipment is delivered and paid for. Upon delivery, test the equipment with the vendor if possible and ask for an in-service with all of your simulation center employees and faculty users on the operation, troubleshooting, and maintenance of the equipment. The final step in the purchasing process is to keep a file that will provide information on the vendor contact information, repairs, replacement, and satisfaction with the entire purchasing experience for reference at a later date.

MANIKINS, TASK TRAINERS, SIMULATORS

No simulation center is complete without patients (manikins), models (task trainers), or clinical simulators. Table 9-1 lists the different types of simulators used by health care educators.

The use of clinical simulators in well-stocked simulation rooms allows for the transformation into a realistic clinical environment. Lifelike manikins, anatomical task trainers, and clinical simulators assist with assessment, problem solving, and critical thinking, as well as the psychomotor skills necessary to prepare students and health care providers to deliver safe and efficient patient care in different health care settings.

Manikins can be tailored to meet individual learner needs and course objectives. Today's clinicians need to be able to provide high-quality care to high acuity and more diverse patient populations. The number of simulators within the simulation center will need to continually reflect the rapid growth of simulation usage, the need for diverse, high acuity experiences, and the ability to replicate various contemporary clinical situations that are just-in-time learning experiences for multiple, diverse learners to facilitate critical thinking, prioritization, and delegation. Some of the most common models available today serve a broad patient population and include the neonate, infant, child, adult, and pregnant female.

When making manikin selections, a center should consider the diversification of the patient population. Advances in manikin development have broadened manikin options to include the ability to present racial, age, and gender differences that are critical for a growing, well-rounded program. In addition, having the ability to modify manikins to fit clinical settings (e.g., trauma or military) is critical when choosing the proper model to gain clinical relevance. Another area to consider is the ability of a manikin to provide live feedback when evaluating learners. One area feedback has proven to be useful is in the operating room where active monitoring of individual performance during anesthesia can be tracked across a spectrum. Another area gaining popularity with live feedback recording is with cardiopulmonary resuscitation (CPR) performance and proficiency testing. As simulation centers increase in size and service more learner types, a center needs the flexibility of wireless manikins for movement from one environment to another which affords the ability to simulate safe handoffs.

Numerous types of task trainers are used to add to the full-body simulator encounter. Incorporating multiple methods of learning will enhance psychomotor skill acquisition, which will lead to skill mastery. The selection of the appropriate simulator is a process of matching the right tool with the right educational objective. Choosing the correct simulator requires an understanding of the strengths, weaknesses, and limitations of each product. A trained technician can walk a faculty member through the process of manikin selection for each simulation scenario. The technician should communicate with the educator to ensure the desired learning outcomes will be met. Another responsibility of the technician should be to provide education about the simulation equipment and manikin capabilities. Task trainers are manufactured by multiple vendors and regardless of the program you are trying to service, there are several factors to consider when purchasing these trainers. These factors include:

- How durable is this product (is it designed for 15 needle insertions or 100)?
- Can it be used in a variety of settings (indoor and outdoor)?
- What is the life expectancy of the manikin (movable parts)?
- Is there a warranty?
- Will the product require servicing? If so, by whom and how often?
- How long is the product expected to last?
- What is the cost of upgrades (software and hardware)?
- Is there any type of special care required (cleaners, adhesive removers)?
- What do the consumable replacement supplies cost?
- Does the product allow for changes in presentation (e.g., Can the pelvic ultrasound model present masses and cysts)?

Clinical simulators carry similar concerns as raised with manikins and task trainers. Some of the biggest concerns that need to be delineated relate to warranties, repair and maintenance, and software and hardware upgrades. One challenge to consider is if another department purchases a simulator and abandons it in the simulation center, who will assume ownership, purchase the next warranty, provide the maintenance, and support the equipment? Although purchased and maintained prior by the owning party, upon transfer of that equipment to the simulation center, the assumption of all upgrades, warranties, and service agreements presents a financial challenge to the simulation center if these type of equipment transfers are not included in the budget planning. The center may find value in obtaining a "letter of understanding" with the individuals loaning or donating the equipment, so both parties understand the terms of agreement and expectations of services following the transition. Unfortunately, these clinical simulators have tremendous and relevant clinical application and no center wants a piece of equipment to become obsolete when simple modifications would have kept it in service for many learners in the future.

Routine care by faculty, learners, and simulation center staff will help maintain and extend the life expectancy of all equipment. The following information includes recommendations to extend the life of manikins and task trainers. The outer surface or skin of a manikin is made of vinyl, latex, flexible or rigid plastic, and fabric. Manikin skins are very sensitive and stain easily. Most manikins are allergic to ink, betadine, some simulated blood products, and many other colored products. In addition, it is not uncommon to need to care for the skin with a multi-stage cleaning process. Any manikin on which an adhesive dressing is applied will need to be cleaned with adhesive remover.

Movable parts and limbs are constructed of hard plastic and metal. The joints and other moveable parts are attached using hinges and other bolt and nut devices. In addition to moveable external parts, some manikins have interchangeable internal parts, which often slide into place via a track and are secured in place with a nut and bolt. Ensure when budgeting ample funds are available for upkeep and replacement of consumable supplies such as lungs, chest rise bladders, tubing, airway structures, and cyanosis pads, among others.

The maintenance, repair, and parts replacement of the manikin will depend on the frequency of use, number and type of moving parts, and the type of simulation skills to be performed. Manikins used for catheterization and rectal examinations may become torn or cracked as a result of frequent internal manipulation. Glue for vinyl and plastic, sutures, and hot pen can be used to repair and reinforce weak and high-stress areas. Replaceable parts often are included with the manikin or available for purchase, such as skin and veins to replace on manikins used for intravenous therapy. As the manikin's parts become unrepairable or replacement parts are no longer available, the need to interchange parts among manikins or modify the intended use of the manikin based on its limitations or capabilities may become necessary. For example, a manikin with destroyed lower legs can become a bilateral amputee patient and this manikin could also be utilized for tracheotomy care, enteral feedings, and other skills where the lower legs are not necessary.

When a repair is required, having the ability to perform diagnostics on the manikin locally may allow you to determine the cause of the problem and have the company ship the repair item to the center and minimize downtime for the manikin. If the manikin is required to be sent out, this can significantly hamper your educational process for extended periods of time if you do not have back-up manikins in your possession. If you are short manikins, then you should contact your local sales representative and determine if a loaner is available until your manikin returns. It is common for a representative to assist in this way depending on the vendor. The more comfortable the manufacturer is with your team, the more likely the repair can be accomplished locally with shipped replacement parts. Maintaining excellent records of all repairs, maintenance schedules, and warranties with renewal dates is very important for monitoring the budget and facilitating to keep the warranties up-to-date. It is recommended to keep a database of all information as it pertains to each piece of equipment.

Although expensive ($30,000 to $170,000), a manikin can last a long time with proper care and preventive maintenance. Equipment and manikins should be stored appropriately; most manufacturers provide a storage unit for each manikin at the time of purchase. Unfortunately, for everyday use, it is impractical to have manikins in their cases and other options are critical to organizing manikin storage. A bunk bed style rolling cart can be a safe storage option for the manikins. Stackable rolling carts provide efficient space usage and can allow ergonomic transportation from the storage room to the bedside by a single person. Storage areas must be dry and cool to prevent manikin damage. An area that is hot and humid may damage internal and external parts. Mildew, mold, spores, and bacteria may grow on and in the manikin even if they are cleaned and thoroughly dried before storage.

SUPPLIES, INVENTORY, AND RESTOCKING

The volume of equipment, supplies, and transactions that are needed for the day-to-day operations of a simulation center necessitate a structured record-keeping program. The inventory system can be written or automated (e.g., barcode or spreadsheet). A planned system will save time and increase accuracy in supply distribution and acquisition. Ideally, a system would provide cross-referencing, automatic notification of low inventory items, notification of routine equipment maintenance and calibration, and generation of reports. No matter what format is selected, one must be able to retrieve information about equipment, manikins, task trainers, special equipment, clinical simulators, and supplies needed, used, or available.

Keeping track of disposable supplies to be used and those already used can be one of the most difficult and time-consuming aspects of the functioning simulation center. The inventory of the equipment can either be formatted by skill (e.g., tracheotomy care), by the type of equipment (e.g, gauze pads, 4 x 4's), or cross-references that allow one to change the format based on the need at the time (e.g., lab setup or review of total equipment available per category). An inventory system spreadsheet contains the item name, description, location in the simulation center, cost, how it is supplied (single, box, case), where to order the supply, how to order the supply (hospital central supply, supply vendor), and an accurate inventory of supplies on hand.

Some inventory management options simulation centers have elected to utilize to maintain records include simple paper and pencil, electronic spreadsheet, bar code system with database, database proper, or a complete scheduling system that incorporates all aspects into a single software system. No matter the system the center employs to maintain records and efficiency, there are multiple departments involved in maintaining adequate supplies in any simulation center. Establishing contacts within the local hospital system can assist in locating expired equipment, consumables, disposables, drug containers, and instruments. Operating rooms are a good place of discarded supplies due to the large number of cases; many stock supplies are pulled for each case in preparation, but if not utilized, the supplies are discarded as trash. When supplies have not had patient or operative field exposure, they can be collected and subsequently recycled to your simulation center, allowing the center and health care system to save on supply costs. It is not uncommon to have a representative at each of the hospital facility operating room units that are looking and collecting these supplies and alerting simulation center leadership when a bag is ready to be picked up. Commonly, there are individuals who donate supplies that have expired or that they no longer need, and these items can be incorporated into all educational events. Vendors commonly will have a set amount of supplies they can donate for educational purposes (e.g., suture, tubing, and lines) that assist in maximizing curricular opportunities. Lastly, many hospital systems have warehouses of expired and outdated supplies and furniture that may have value. Learn where the system maintains this warehouse and schedule a visit; it may contain something useful for your center.

Restocking is a critical and time consuming task for simulation center staff. Once supply orders are filled, they need to be placed in storage locations. This takes vital time away from a technician's day and limits their ability to service customers, either running, developing, or programming simulations. Look within your system to determine if you have the ability to automate this process. If allowed, take advantage of the hospital system supply chain and all of its amenities. Utilizing the standard hospital restocking system with par levels for all supplies, self-stocking of the simulation center shelves by hospital personnel, and automated billing for the supplies consumed is most convenient. By establishing par levels, the center will never have more supplies than the storage system can tolerate. When an event may require a large volume of a set of supplies, an order can be placed in advance for that event and delivered via the hospital system. This pulls all simulation center staff from maintaining any supplies considered standard and allows them to dedicate time to higher priority tasks. A second area of efficiency is utilizing volunteers within your system to assist with supply related activities. There are many volunteer systems within the medical community that often are willing to regularly schedule one or more volunteers. But keep in mind they will need guidance and supervision.

Plan to recycle as much as possible. Many disposable items can be reused in the simulation environment before they become fatigued and unusable. Recycling and reusing will require some ingenuity and engineering, but the cost savings are worth the effort. Items to reuse multiple times include nasogastric tubes, urinary catheters, defibrillation pads, refilled intravenous fluid bags, intravenous fluid tubing and connectors, central venous catheters, oxygen adjuncts, drug vials, and injection devices. Before disposing of equipment, always ask the question, "Can this item be repurposed?" or "Will this work for another purpose?" Customers will frequently request a type of commonly utilized medical equipment in their simulation scenario, if real items are not available upon request, then a creative challenge exists to meet the needs of that simulation. Preparation and ordering the equipment ahead of time before the simulation is run is important so a high quality simulation is developed and implemented.

SCHEDULING

The day-to-day functions of the simulation center depend on an organized scheduling system that can account for center rooms, equipment resources, learner data, and personnel availability. An organized scheduling system will prevent a learner group from arriving unexpectedly and minimize the occurrences of multiple groups not having appropriate space for their number of learners.

A block time schedule may work well for some customers, while open access with flexibility works better for others. The manner in which a center's time is allotted depends on the customer and uses. A goal of a simulation center is to project the schedule prior to the start of a fiscal or academic year. Unfortunately, there is no ideal world in the simulation center, as new classes are added, customers are recruited, learner needs change, and tours and presentations with the community occur without warning. Although there is always an unpredictable aspect to the simulation center, one can work to establish a calendar of "big events" to avoid major conflicts.

Simulation center scheduling of activities and durable equipment, supplies, personnel, and other information will always be a challenge when trying to meet the requests of customers. There are a few software systems on the market; however, all of them are in their early phases of development and implementation. Many systems have developed local, home-grown software systems or are utilizing less sophisticated processes. These less sophisticated processes have been tolerated in the past due to the relatively small size of most simulation centers and the predictable number of learner groups for that system. However, with new simulation centers being built throughout the world, few of them have the small footprint of past centers. With the increased size, complexity, number of personnel, and the fact that these centers are run as sophisticated businesses, software solutions are critical. One can approach scheduling through a coordinator or technician (manually), but this will require one or two key personnel to schedule all aspects of the center's use. This would be recorded on some form of calendar. Another method is to utilize an electronic or web-based system that allows real-time scheduling that is visible to the user. This will allow for an electronic copy of the request to be saved and housed within system in the event of lost or mistaken data. This also will allow for confirmation notices to be sent alerting educators of all specific reservation data for their event. Some centers will use multiple scheduling systems before they find the best fit for their environment. Table 9-6 includes items that might be important to consider when selecting a software system.

Table 9-6 Selecting a Software System
• Online capabilities for customer registration, the ability to request time and place, and for an event request to placed into the scheduling software
• Multiple status levels for request order (preliminary, reviewed, active, cancelled, invoiced)
• Ability to schedule all rooms associated
• Ability to schedule all equipment
• Ability to schedule all supplies
• Have journaling entries to follow communication thread
• Allow for invoicing
• Allow for complete reporting
• Allow for online payments of services
• Project management software to assign tasks and communicate needs
• Maintain full customer database and contact information
• Provide database for statistical tracking of customer base, research, and competencies evaluation
• Provide online calendar and room availability for customers
• Have multi-user platform

Examples of a simulation center reservation form, whether submitted online, via email or in writing, can be seen in Table 9-7.

Table 9-7 Sample Reservation Form Items
1. Name, contact information, affiliation
2. Event title, purpose, objectives
3. Learner group and numbers of participants
4. Date requested, times, and other optional dates
5. Rooms requested
6. Equipment desired
7. Personnel required
8. Supplies desired

It is critical for any system to have the ability to recognize conflicts. These conflicts might include rooms, equipment, supplies, or technician availability. One example that may occur is when a customer requests two ventilators for use in a simulation and the center only has one available. The software should alert scheduling staff of the equipment conflict, which will then allow the system to locate a second ventilator or work with the customer to adjust the simulation event to stagger the use of the ventilator so all aspects of the scenario can be maintained.

STRATEGIC PLANNING

There is a tremendous amount of excitement and stress that go into the planning, implementing, and eventual opening of the doors of a new center. Strategic planning should involve all levels of leadership, from the executive committee down to the operational group. It is not uncommon to have a one-year, three-year, five-year, or longer outlook to act as a system compass. Goals, objectives, and metrics should be established and tracked for success and failures (Gantt, 2010).

OUTREACH

Initially, increasing the awareness and knowledge of the simulation center's presence within the health care system and community at large is critical to attract participants for programs and future donors. This can be accomplished by electronic communication, an active, thriving website, invitations to courses and events within the center, utilization of media sources (video, text, newspapers, and magazines), alumni and special events, open houses, tours, school events, hosting students, and the distribution of brochures. Large centers should prepare to conduct hundreds of tours each year for various members of the health care system and schools. This takes a tremendous amount of resources and most centers will have difficulty determining which tour will have an impact on the future of the center. Keep in mind that if you touch just one person with the passion you carry every day, it will have been a successful tour and the future will remain bright for assistance and support.

A dedicated website that can represent the center as a state-of-the-art facility within the system is critical and can be utilized for many aspects of center function. The site needs to serve as the face of the simulation center to entities that support the center's development and the public at large. If it is functional and offers resources to others, the site will thrive and drive new initiatives. The site should house basic information with location and directions, contact information, key individuals, information on scheduling, services offered, faculty information, courses offered, virtual tours, pictures of center and floor plan, calendar of room use, educational resources, donation and volunteering opportunities, references, current news and upcoming meetings, research information, standard operating procedures, mission, vision, objectives of the center, resources available within the center, and a database of scenarios and equipment.

As simulation center users quickly adopt this method of teaching and evaluation into their practice, expect many different forms of requests. Some decisions can be made by the leadership team before these requests start arriving. Below is a list of frequently asked questions by outreach customers.

- Will the center loan equipment to customers for off-site use?
- Will the center bring a manikin to the clinical unit where our staff and learners practice?
- Can my child's school visit for a tour and interact with the manikins?

Additional Design and Operations Standards

The success of a simulation center can be ensured by considering accreditation needs of the organizations involved and incorporating best practices and standards employed by organizations committed to advancing the use of simulation in health care practice such as the Society for Simulation in Healthcare (SSH). The SSH Council for Accreditation of Healthcare Simulation Programs has developed core standards for organizations using simulation technologies and methodologies in health care education. The SSH core standards include mission and governance, organization and management, facilities, application and technology, evaluation and improvement, integrity, and expanding the field. The SSH also provides additional standards and criteria for the areas of assessment, research, teaching and education, system integrating, and patient safety standards (Society for Simulation in Healthcare, 2012).

Summary

Fidelity or realism is one of the key design characteristics that should be included in every simulation. This chapter emphasizes the key components of the simulation center environment necessary to enhance the teaching strategy and the learners' ability to achieve the desired curriculum outcomes. The selection of equipment, supplies, simulators, and personnel are integral to bringing the vision alive and transforming the center's environment into a realistic replication of the clinical setting. This is accentuated by the efficient and effective day-to-day operations and management of the center.

The design of a simulation area that realistically reflects the clinical practice environment will help learners and practicing health care providers to be safer and more efficient within the patient environment. Faced with the challenges of today's health care environment, all educators must explore innovative ways to teach learners about the real world in a cost-effective, efficient, and high-quality manner. The simulated environment provides a setting in which the learner can actively engage in the learning process and receive immediate feedback from educators. The simulation center has been designed with the right blend of simulators that allow learners to experience and practice in an environment where mistakes result in teachable moments and not patient morbidity and mortality. This learning does not always happen without anxiety; however, clinical simulation, combined with clinical experiences and other teaching methods, is a powerful tool to prepare competent health care providers for clinical practice.

REFERENCES

American College of Surgeons (2012). *How to become accredited.* In http://www.facs.org. Retrieved April 15, 2012, from http://www.facs.org/education/accreditationprogram/application.html.

Gantt, L. T. (2010). Strategic planning for skills and simulation labs in colleges of nursing. *Nursing Economics, 28*(5), 308-313.

Hyland, J. R., & Hawkins, M. C. (2009). High fidelity human simulation in nursing education: A review of the literature and guide for implementation. *Teaching and Learning in Nursing, 4*(1), 14-21.

Infante, M.S. (1985). *The clinical laboratory in nursing education* (2nd ed.). New York: John Wiley.

Kardong-Edgren, S., & Oermann, M. (2009). A letter to nursing program administrators about simulation. *Clinical Simulations in Nursing, 5*(5), e161-e162.

Seropian, M., & Lavey, R. (2010). Design considerations for healthcare simulation facilities. *The Journal of the Society for Simulation in Healthcare, 5*(6), 338-345.

Society for Simulation in Healthcare. (2012). Accreditation Program. In *www.ssih.org* . Retrieved April 19, 2012, from https://ssih.org/accreditation-of-health care-simulation-programs.

CHAPTER 10
USING COLLABORATION TO ENHANCE THE EFFECTIVENESS
OF SIMULATED LEARNING IN NURSING EDUCATION

Julie McAfooes, MS, RN-BC, CNE, ANEF
Reba Moyer Childress, MSN, RN, FNP, FAANP, ANEF
Pamela R. Jeffries, PhD, RN, FAAN, ANEF
Cheryl Feken, MS, RN

"Part of teaching is helping students learn how to tolerate ambiguity, consider possibilities, and ask questions that are unanswerable."

–Sara Lawrence Lightfoot

Nursing, like many other professions, has used diverse educational methods to guide student learning to help students become safe and effective clinicians. Traditionally, the methods have been teacher-centered and focused primarily on the cognitive domain (e.g., lectures, seminars, and discussions). However, faculty are finding more effective ways to prepare today's students to care for patients who are more acutely ill, to manage the care of increasing numbers of patients, and to practice in high-tech, fast-paced clinical environments.

With the advancement of technology, the demands on health care providers have become more complex (Bonnell & Vogel Smith, 2010). Health care providers face challenging patient care situations, the need to make decisions rapidly in spite of conflicting or incomplete information, and the need to collaborate more effectively among members of the health care team (Hamman, 2004; Maddox, Wakefield, & Bull, 2001). Such realities drive or force nurse educators and others in the health professions to design teaching, learning, and evaluation strategies that enhance students' abilities to practice safely and effectively in this health care environment. Among the strategies suggested to assist educators in meeting student learning needs and developing their practice competencies through collaborative learning is through the use of various teaching strategies such as e-learning, virtual reality, and scenario-based simulations (Skiba, Conners, & Jeffries, 2009; Ziv, Wolpe, Small, & Glick, 2003). Collaborative learning using scenario-based simulation holds exceptional promise for education, particularly for the education of nurses.

Collaboration in health care education increasingly refers to the development of interprofessional partnerships among nurses and other disciplines. In 2010, the Institute of Medicine (IOM) released its landmark report *The Future of Nursing: Leading Change, Advancing Health.* The IOM recommended that "schools of nursing, in collaboration with other health professional schools, should design and implement early and continuous interprofessional collaboration through joint classroom and clinical training opportunities" (2010, p. 4). This IOM report has provided momentum to integrate simulation into health care education as an effective means to facilitate students' acquisition of psychomotor skills, decision-making skills, and skills related to collaborating with other members of the health care team (Loyd, Lake, & Greenberg, 2004).

The Interprofessional Education Collaborative (IPEC), comprised of experts across multiple health care disciplines, developed 38 essential core competencies under four domains for interprofessional collaborative practice (Interprofessional Education Collaborative Expert Panel, 2011).

Competency Domain 1: Values/Ethics stresses competencies about working with other professions in an environment of respect. *Competency Domain 2: Roles/Responsibilities* highlights the need to understand how roles and responsibilities complement each other. *Competency Domain 3: Interprofessional Communication* speaks to communication not only with other health professionals but also individuals, families, and communities.

Finally, *Competency Domain 4: Teams and Teamwork* describes how team dynamics and relationship building contribute to planning and carrying out patient- or population-centered care. The expert panel recognizes the value of students from different professions learning interactively with each other.

Collaborative efforts by the Society for Simulation in Healthcare and the National League for Nursing (NLN) have fueled partnerships among stakeholders in health care education who are also interested in interprofessional education, to discover their unique perspectives, best practices in the use of simulation for interprofessional education (IPE), knowledge gaps, research needs, and future collaboration opportunities (NLN, 2011). The collaborative, sponsored by a grant from the Josiah Macy Jr. Foundation, included key representatives from 24 organizations representing health professions education, practice, accreditation, and patient safety. The outcomes of this teamwork have the potential to dramatically impact health care education though the promotion of simulation-based interprofessional education.

This chapter defines collaborative learning in a health care simulation environment by describing different types of collaborative learning experiences that can be incorporated into a simulation. It identifies roles faculty may participate in when designing a simulation with an emphasis on collaboration, discusses benefits and challenges associated with incorporating collaborative learning in a simulated environment, and forecasts future trends for collaboration through simulation.

COLLABORATIVE LEARNING DEFINED

Collaborative learning in a simulated health care environment is defined as the process of individuals functioning together as a group for the purpose of acquiring knowledge and skills to improve individual and team performance, as well as improve patient outcomes. Working together results in greater understanding that would not have occurred had each person worked independently. Team members are assigned to or assume various roles, have a common objective, and function in a simulated health care setting to achieve common goals (Freeth et al., 2009). Through interactive experiences both in and beyond the classroom, collaborative learners forge relationships using interactions which lead to deeper understanding about the learner and patient outcomes.

ESTABLISHING A COLLABORATIVE LEARNING ENVIRONMENT

In all disciplines, learning involves induction into the intellectual culture of the discipline (Hamilton, 1997). For example, to understand anthropology, students need to learn how anthropologists look at people and events. To enact the role of a historian, anthropologist, physician, or nurse, students need appropriate information, language, and experiences. Also, opportunities need to be developed through which learners can connect the information, language, and experiences to their own knowledge and experience to ensure understanding. Lectures, laboratory experiences, and videos are learning tools that foster efficient and rapid delivery of essential information or development of specialized skills or techniques. However, unless students apply this knowledge and these skills to the context of work done by individuals in the field, the skills, knowledge, and information may be forgotten. As students are involved in health care problem solving and decision-making, they need to integrate information, language, and skills into action and dialogue. As students become immersed in this type of learning environment, they can solve problems together and gain a better understanding of roles and responsibilities specific to each discipline.

Deciding when to use collaborative learning is dependent upon the nature of the knowledge and understanding expected in a particular area. Facts, standardized skills, and interventions are efficiently learned in a lecture format. Application of new information and new skills in response to less predictable real-life situations is more effectively accomplished in a collaborative atmosphere in which students can interact and integrate knowledge and skills in a realistic manner.

Virtual learning environments have made it possible for health care students to safely engage in simulated learning experiences during the same time, but not necessarily in the same place. Simulation need not be bound by physical settings. Instead, the internet provides virtual space for students to meet, analyze, and apply information, thus removing the barrier to collaboration and learning that is caused by distance.

The University of Michigan School of Nursing recently developed a new strategy in educating nursing students utilizing the asynchronous, Internet-based program Second Life® (Abersold, Tschannen, Stephens, Anderson, & Lei,2011). This innovative, computer-based program was designed and implemented utilizing a virtual hospital unit and was pilot tested with 15 students and three scenarios that focused on patient safety, as well as key student learning challenges. Students participating in the experience completed an evaluation survey and reported that they had benefited from the experience. The virtual shared environment can provide students a space to interact, problem solve, and complete assignments. The experience of a professional community can be created through the Second Life platform and may provide students the ability to interact and collaborate with other health care professionals in interprofessional learning experiences.

The members of the European Union (EU) recognized the value of using virtual patients (VPs) in medical and health care education, but noted that it took considerable time and resources to develop VPs and that there was much duplication of effort (Zary et al., 2009). The EU has funded the standardization of VP design and implementation to promote interoperability, accessibility, and reusability of VPs across Europe. The European

Virtual Patient Project (eViP) is an example of how nine universities are working together in a collaborative manner to break down barriers to use simulations in a virtual environment.

COLLABORATIVE LEARNING EXPERIENCES IN HEALTH PROFESSIONS EDUCATION

Types of collaborative learning experiences that can be designed in a simulation are variable and involve many different disciplines, practice settings, and health care scenarios. Examples of collaborative learning in health care settings are described below and summarized in Table 10-1.

Table 10-1 Types of Collaborative Learning Experiences	
Type	Description
Student-to-Student	Student learners or peers support one another's acquisition of knowledge and skills as a team.
Faculty-to-Student	Through teacher-learner interactions, students gain direction and validation from the expert.
Academic Faculty-to-Clinicians/ Clinical Faculty	Academic faculty in the simulated clinical setting collaborates with clinicians in health care settings to establish pre-clinical and alternative clinical learning experience for students.
Interdisciplinary	Students from various disciplines learn together to manage various health care situations as a team, identify appropriate responsibilities for each role, and develop mutual respect for the contribution each makes to the team.

Student-to-Student

In student-to-student collaboration, student learners, or peers, support one another's acquisition of knowledge and skills as a team. An example of this type of collaborative learning would be students practicing in pairs to learn how to take a blood pressure reading in preparation for a clinical demonstration. Wright (2003) provided a collaborative learning experience for nursing students in an environmental health class by pairing undergraduate students with graduate students from the school of public health. The 190 participants in the study concluded that the collaborative process was helpful. The group activities on environmental issues demonstrated how nursing students could function as members of a professional team, and knowledge of the environmental issues increased significantly ($p > .05$) after the collaborative activity. On the down side, however, this type of student-to-student collaboration can have a higher risk of not succeeding if the experience is driven by novices or is limited in faculty direction. For student-to-student collaboration to be successful, it also is important to match individuals' learning styles (Brewer, 2011). Students are individuals with diverse learning styles. Fountain and Alfred (2009) conducted a study using a convenience sample of 76 baccalaureate students. The investigation compared social learning style to solitary learning and examined whether student learning style had an influence on the satisfaction level associated with a patient simulation experience. Results revealed that 76 percent of the students preferred social learning style, whereby listening, networking, comparing, and interacting with other students were a major focus of the experience. A limitation of this study was small sample size and that only descriptive data were collected, which may have resulted in group perception.

Faculty-to-Student

Faculty members are in a unique position to help motivate and shape students (Chickering & Gamson, 1987). Through teacher-learner interactions such as simulated patient rounds by a group of health care students and the instructor, students can gain direction and validation from the expert. This support can encourage students to proceed in the learning process even when they encounter academic obstacles. In addition, students' values and belief systems are shaped through these types of relationships. In professional schools, such as nursing, it is important for faculty and students to recognize that students are not only scholars or learners, but also future colleagues, who will one day serve as mentors themselves (Childress, 2005). When objectives and goals are provided, the faculty-to-student pattern of interaction tends to have a greater success rate for active learning than student-to-student (Murphy, Hartigan, Walshe, Flynn, & O'Brien, 2011; Wotton, Davis, Button, & Kelton, 2010).

Academic Faculty-to-Clinicians or Clinical Faculty

Academic faculty in the simulated clinical setting facilitate collaboration with clinicians in health care settings by establishing experiences for students prior to entering the clinical setting. Also, the virtual learning center can be used as an alternative learning environment for students who need additional experiences to help master process, integrate theory with practice in the clinical setting, manage patient care situations, and learn how to interact with patients and other health care professionals as a team. One example of this type of collaborative learning experience is incorporating simulations into clinical orientations. Another example is an academic faculty member working in the simulation setting with students who need additional help to master clinical skills, while the clinical faculty member remains on the clinical unit with the other students. This model considers learners' needs and allows all learners to proceed at their own pace. It also provides a clinical group with the opportunity to continue their clinical experience in the simulation center.

Interprofessional

It is important when creating simulation scenarios to include professionals from a variety of health care disciplines. This model helps students to identify appropriate responsibilities for each role and develop mutual respect for the contribution of each member of the health care team. Students from various disciplines (e.g., nursing and medical students, first-responders, and others) come together to learn how to manage resuscitation emergencies, terrorist events, rescue efforts, and routine health care situations. For example, Reese, Jeffries, and Engum (2010) conducted a study placing third-year medical students with senior nursing students to help them learn how to work together to provide care for a post-operative patient. The medical and nursing students worked together in a 20-minute simulation followed by a 20-minute debriefing. The patient in the scenario was a post-operative adult who developed acute chest pain, multi-focal premature ventricular contractions (PVC)s, and eventual ventricular tachycardia. The learning outcomes measured in the study included teamwork, collaboration, and interdisciplinary communication.

In a recent study, faculty in the University of Mary Hardin-Baylor BSN program developed and implemented a multidisciplinary, collaborative, high-fidelity simulation involving graduating senior nursing students and internal medicine residents (Booth & McMullen-Fix, 2012). Common objectives were developed for both teams that focused on safe clinical practice, effective interprofessional communication, and implementation of appropriate decision-making in the management of multiple patients. Results of this experience reinforce that the role of simulation is important to improve interprofessional communication, and enhance awareness of safety when caring for multiple patients.

GOALS IN A COLLABORATIVE LEARNING ENVIRONMENT

In collaborative learning, the educator and students share goal setting. In the case of a simulation, the goals students desire to achieve from the simulation and the goals the educator hopes to meet both need to be considered.

Goals of the Educator

During a collaborative experience such as a simulation, the educator may desire that students understand interventions and problem solving pertaining to the care of a specific client and health disruption or a specific goal as described in the course syllabus. Whatever the goal, the educator generally has an outcome in mind. For example, the educator may have the goal that students are able to identify a basic arrhythmia and implement priority interventions to care for a patient experiencing this disorder. Goals with predictable answers are discussed in the debriefing sessions following the simulation. Open-ended goals have several avenues of inquiry that could produce a variety of unpredictable responses; open-ended goals usually motivate more lateral thinking and more widespread participation among group members. The achievement of this type of goal can also be accomplished in debriefing sessions or in the classroom.

Goals of the Learner

Learners should formulate their own goals based on the collaborative teaching-learning activity they plan to encounter. When students perceive that they are working to achieve their own goals as well as the educator's goals, they are more committed to the work of the simulation and the course (Hamilton, 1997). Students sharing their goals in a group help other group members with their goal achievement. Educators at times may need to assist students with their goal setting, since the goals will affect the nature of inquiry and activity within the simulated experience.

TOOLS FOR COLLABORATION

Communication is often identified as the primary root of errors in patient care (Enlow, Shanks, Guhde, & Perkins, 2010). Accurate and effective communication between health care students and professionals is imperative to patient safety. Communication between and among health care students and professionals can be complex, depending on the nature of patient care, level or complexity of technology, changing and increasing standards of care, and enforcement by regulatory agencies (Thomas, Bertram, & Johnson, 2009).

The Joint Commission's (TJC) (2010) Patient Safety Advisory Group reported 802 sentinel events related to patient safety in 2010. The number of events increased to 914 for January to September 30, 2011 (TJC, 2011). The Agency for Healthcare Research and Quality (AHRQ) and TJC recommended the use of standardized communication in health care facilities to improve patient safety (Enlow et al., 2010; TJC, 2008). Communication errors can be attributed to multiple organizational and environmental factors such as frequent interruptions and extraneous noises within the environment. The increased patient acuity can lead to too much information resulting in cognitive overload and the inability to make decisions. Two-way, face-to-face, written communication tools have been found to have vital components and content that capture the receiver's attention (Jukkala, 2012). Incorporating interprofessional communication simulations into curricula can prepare learners to communicate effectively with other health care professionals, which can lead to improved patient safety (Margalit et al., 2009). The Agency for Health Research and Quality (AHRQ, n.d.) has developed TeamSTEPPS™ as an evidence-based teamwork system to improve patient safety through communication. The American Institutes for Research prepared a training guide for AHRQ to help instructors use simulation to teach TeamSTEPPS. The guide highlights the power of simulation to enhance the quality of continuing education for health professionals.

Another communication tool widely used in nursing education is the SBAR (situation, background, assessment, recommendation), which recently was reformulated to ISBARR (introduction, situation, background, assessment, recommendation, and readback) (Grbach, Vincent, & Struth, 2008). ISBARR helps promote a brief, organized, and predictable flow of information about a patient's condition. The organized information allows other health care providers to make clinical judgments based on the concrete information provided (Thomas, Bertram, & Johnson, 2009). Quality and Safety Education for Nurses (QSEN) includes ISBARR as a tool for communication and teaching strategies for implementation with the goal to improve the quality and safety of patient care (Grbach et al.).

FACULTY ROLES IN COLLABORATIVE LEARNING SIMULATION EXPERIENCES

During a collaborative learning simulation experience, a faculty member may function in a variety of roles in the teaching-learning environment as depicted in Table 10-2. Smith-Stoner (2009) described the role of instructors in an end-of-life simulation scenario running the simulator and equipment. She stated a second instructor acted as a standardized actor and assumed the role of the spouse. Reid, Sinclair, and Hudson (2011) described multidisciplinary simulations providing an opportunity for interprofessional teamwork, education, and pro-active patient management discussions and practice changes. The co-facilitated, instructor-led debriefing sessions explored the experience of participants and provoked reflective practice to identify areas of learning, clinical strengths, and areas requiring remediation.

Table 10-2 Faculty Roles When Using Simulations in Nursing Education	
Role	Description
Patient or Other Member of the Care Team	Provides authenticity and consistency in the learning process
Facilitator	Guides but does not dictate the learning experience
Debriefer	Provides opportunities for students to reflect on what worked well and areas for improvement; faculty provides expert knowledge during this process
Evaluator	Provides progress report on development of competence
Researcher	Seeks to answer questions regarding the use of simulation in nursing education

Patient or Other Member of the Care Team

In the role as standardized patient, the faculty member takes on the characteristics and physical condition of a particular patient so students may have an opportunity to practice and refine certain skills. For example, the faculty member could assume the role of an ailing geriatric client (including appearance and behaviors consistent with the script) from whom the student learner must obtain a health history. As a standardized patient, faculty may provide more authenticity to the situation because of their professional knowledge and experience (Anderson, 2010). Although assuming this role may be time-consuming, it may minimize the costs of recruiting and training lay individuals to play the role. In addition, faculty members as standardized patients may be able to give a more consistent simulated learning experience as it is presented to each student. This, in turn, may improve students' acquisition of knowledge and skills.

The faculty member also might be assigned to the role of care team member. Johnson, Zerwic, and Theis (1999) assigned a faculty member to the role of a physician, where she or he would periodically receive phone calls from students who reported on a particular patient and conditions or problems. Again, the faculty member's expertise makes it possible to take on such a role quite effectively.

Facilitator

In the facilitator role, the faculty member serves as a guide rather than as a teacher; he or she is not directly dictating what learners need to do or determining a particular sequence the learners should use, but rather supporting the objectives for the collaborative learning experience. These objectives are used to guide or assist the students in working as a group when completing the simulation experience. When constructing a simulation scenario, it is important to provide students with a situation that requires them to utilize each other and to solve problems as a team. Providing opportunities for problem solving challenges students to examine personal perceptions of knowledge, to rely on each other to provide information, to establish a different view or framework based on exposure to diverse interpretations of available information, and to formulate a cooperative plan as to how to proceed as a group to solve the situation (Smith & MacGregor, 1992). One example of faculty taking on the role of facilitator is giving a simulation case study to a group of students and allowing them time to work through the problem of caring for the patient during a set time frame while the faculty member is present in the room but not available to direct the process.

Debriefer

Once the simulation learning experience has been implemented, the learning experience is not complete until the students and faculty member have had an opportunity to reflect on the implementation process. During the reflection phase, students (and faculty) have the opportunity to identify how or whether decision-making was appropriate, as well as what areas need improvement. In the debriefer role, faculty members help students identify areas within the simulation where they did well, provide instruction for areas that have gaps, and provide students with support that will allow them to move forward in the learning process. Faculty in the role of debriefer provide novice learners or clinicians with expert knowledge and guidance. For example, students functioning in a mock code may be able to implement all the necessary steps to provide recovery for the patient, but they may not recognize that some of the steps should have been implemented in a different sequence to improve the effectiveness of their actions. The debriefing process after the simulation provides an opportunity for learners to reflect on the process or until the expert shares this information with them during the reflective thinking process. In the debriefing, students can also actively build upon prior learning and test assumptions about patient care and subsequent responses with the other participants in the simulation experience through encouragement of the clinical instructor (Dreifuerst, 2009).

Evaluator

An important piece of the learning process is evaluation. It is important to assess and document competencies and skill sets. Students need feedback to determine whether or not they are on the right track. Validation is also needed to ensure safety of clients. Simulations can help teach theory and develop problem solving and clinical reasoning skills. Simulations also help assess a student's performance progress when the simulation has been designed to measure competence (Salas & Burke, 2002; Satish & Streufert, 2002). It is important that faculty members in the role of evaluator help the novice acquire knowledge and appropriate behavioral skills.

BENEFITS AND CHALLENGES OF COLLABORATIVE LEARNING IN SIMULATED EXPERIENCES

It is important to note that collaborative learning is an excellent way to foster student learning. Students and faculty have important roles to play in the collaborative learning process. There are several benefits and challenges that need to be addressed when considering incorporating collaborative learning experiences in simulation education.

Benefits of collaborative learning

The benefits of health care students learning in collaborative environments are varied and many. Interprofessional training is recognized as an important and formative experience for health care students and professionals with respect to patient safety and quality of care.

Interprofessional simulations provide the opportunity for participants to understand the various roles, skills, and expectations while appreciating the value each member of the health care team contributes to the achievement of common goals. Health care students share common core values, knowledge, and skills typically taught in isolation and specific to their discipline. This can result in these learners building their professional identities based on power, competition, and hierarchies, resulting in inadequate preparation for teamwork. These learners are then unrealistically expected to function in integrated and interdependent health care teams.

The interprofessional educational approach helps the learner identify the contribution each discipline makes in providing patient care. Learning collaboratively in interdisciplinary teams, health care students can develop respectful and effective communication, and increase understanding of roles while promoting better patient outcomes (Dillon, Noble, & Kaplan, 2009). As students work together to care for a patient in a collaborative simulated environment, they learn the responsibilities of other disciplines, as well as how to function as a team member. Feedback from the educator or facilitator allows for more specific assessment of learning achievements and helps identify areas in which more knowledge and practice may be needed individually or as a team.

Another benefit of group learning is the achievement of higher levels of thought, a deeper understanding of content, and the ability to retain information longer than students who work individually (Johnson & Johnson, 1986). In addition, cooperative learning experiences provide opportunities for students to work together as a team to apply knowledge gained in the classroom setting, to solve problems through discussion and reflection, and to develop critical thinking abilities (Gokhale, 1995; Rau & Heyl, 1990). Such experiences also assist them in coping with anxiety associated with the learning process (Gokhale), help them learn professional collaborative skills while working together, and improve confidence.

Collaborative learning experiences motivate students and promote active learning. Active learning, a principle of best practices in education (Chickering & Gamson, 1987), encourages students to engage in the learning activities, focuses on developing students' abilities and skills during the process, provides opportunities that allow students to explore attitudes and values, increases student motivation to learn, provides opportunities for immediate feedback from the instructor, and fosters analytical thinking. Collaborative simulated learning provides a means of bridging the learning gap between generations. Incorporating collaborative learning experiences in simulation can provide students an opportunity to enhance their critical thinking through inclusion of problem solving situations.

A simulated health care setting can provide an ideal active learning environment that is safe, engaging, and realistic. Health care simulation scenarios (e.g., mock codes or resuscitation events) can be developed to allow students to work in teams. When functioning in a group, students work together to solve problems and provide care during the simulated experience. During the group experience, students also have the opportunity to support each other during stressful situations. In this collaborative learning experience, students can reflect and analyze together what worked effectively and share ideas about areas where improvement may be necessary. Working in groups helps students learn from each other, as well as develop and hone decision-making and critical-thinking skills. Fuhrmann and Zambrana (2010) reported that a multidisciplinary perinatal team developed an assessment tool that showed an increase in communication skills among team members after participation in simulated emergent situations.

Simulation allows students to assimilate isolated pieces of data and discern pertinent information from irrelevant information. Simulation activities also invite students to participate in groups when the learning experience is designed with this goal in mind. Sharing patient data helps them develop decision-making skills with decreased stress (Gokhale, 1995), as students are more comfortable sharing ideas in a group than in a faculty-student situation. When in groups, concepts can be clarified and problem solving implemented among peers and clinical instructors more easily than in a one-on-one situation with a clinical instructor. In addition, students have the opportunity to see how others solve problems.

Benefits to collaborative relationships between schools and institutions include the sharing of equipment and resources. In an era when educational institutions are experiencing decreased appropriations, sharing of equipment and resources is a positive investment for all agencies. Free-standing simulation centers that are not affiliated with any one particular institution have been created to serve the needs of many users in a region. One example is the Keystone Simulation & Education Center (KSEC, n.d.) in Monaca, Pennsylvania. This 24,000-square-foot facility provides educational experiences for those who cannot afford to equip and manage state-of-the-art simulation centers. Its simulated emergency room, ambulance, birthing suite, neonatal intensive care unit, pharmacy, blood bank, medical-surgical unit, and other areas educate health care students and staff.

Challenges of collaborative learning

Challenges associated with collaborative simulated learning include having adequate and appropriate simulation equipment to promote active learning (Booth & McMullen-Fix, 2012). Collaborative learning does not facilitate individual learning styles, and buy-in for group learning needs to occur, especially from those who tend to be more individual learners. Another limitation is having adequate time to implement the simulation, including provision of instructions, the actual simulation, debriefing, and incorporating simulations into programs and courses. Other considerations that must be made include the following:

Individual learning styles

Gokhale (1995) examined the effectiveness of individual learning versus collaborative learning in enhancing drill-and-practice skills and critical-thinking skills. In a core collaborative learning environment, individual differences become part of the rich culture of the group rather than a detriment to any member of the group. By implementing a variety of teaching strategies appropriate to content, settings, learner needs, learning style, and desired learning outcomes, faculty have the potential to increase the overall learning of students (Fink, 2009).

Learning silos

Lencioni (2006) defined professional silos as "the barriers that exist between departments within an organization that cause people who are supposed to be on the same team to work against one another" (p. 175). Educators are well aware professional silos exist in educational and health care settings, and these silos adversely affect patient safety. Silos result in fragmented patient care, medical errors, and professional frustration that affects communication. The focus on patient-centered care has increased the need to break down learning silos in order for health professionals to learn from and with each other in real-life settings (Robertson & Bandali, 2008). However, removing the silos of traditional isolated learning in academic and care institutions is a significant barrier to overcome. Institutions will have to engage in curriculum redesign, which will require educational institutions to evaluate issues of cost, scheduling, and utilization of faculty. Simulation provides a risk-free, positive learning environment to practice communication, conflict resolution, and teamwork among various professional groups. Communication problems have been a major cause of patient safety problems and in response the Joint Commission (TJC) has developed National Patient Safety Goals (TJC, 2011). One goal is to improve the effectiveness of communication among caregivers. A way to pursue this goal is to encourage team training, which some schools are accomplishing through interdisciplinary simulation.

Leveling of students

Novice students benefit from sharing ideas and processing situations with each other. In addition, they need experts to help them gain insight into situations that are unfamiliar to them. An advanced provider such as a nurse-practitioner or physician can assist the inexperienced learner to apply techniques such as SBAR (situation, background, assessment, recommendation) communication. These experienced health care professionals can explain how to integrate findings and develop recommendations for the care of individuals.

Matching leveling or learner capabilities is important to consider, as there may be concern about the additional time needed to bring less capable peers along. If the collaborative learning experience is structured so that all students are required to participate, then all can give help within the group as well as receive it. In this way, students of all abilities and different learning styles can work together effectively.

Group selection

The level and type of student participating in the collaborative learning experience can improve participation and learning outcomes. There is a possibility, however, that some students may be more intellectually mature than others and this may cause frustration if students such as these are expected to bear more group responsibilities than other students. According to Gokhale's (1995) research on relationships between collaborative learning and critical thinking, some students found too much time was spent explaining material to group members. In a recent study investigating the benefit of collaborative learning, researchers found that teamwork can benefit students by enhancing their ability to think critically, solve problems creatively, and collaborate effectively (Yang, Woomer, & Matthews, 2012).

Group size

Group size must promote active participation of team members and allow the group to maintain time on task and use time efficiently. Nehring, Lashley, and Ellis (2002) found that simulation groups larger than eight to 10 students prevented students from adequately observing and interacting with the patient and simulation equipment.

Cost

Simulation design and development are initially time consuming and can be costly, depending on the degree of realism. The cost of mannequins, props, and other resources can be overwhelming. Various partnerships can help reduce these expenses. Costs may be borne by one institution but recovered by allowing other departments or institutions to use the resources for a fee. Some schools of nursing have already implemented this type of arrangement. Developing partnerships with agencies that have products necessary for student simulation learning is invaluable when designing and developing simulation programs.

Synchronicity

Collaborative learning in simulated environments requires synchronizing the time and the place for faculty and students to gather. As the diversity of the group increases, so do the difficulties in scheduling all the key players who must be present for the simulated learning experience.

One way to address the problem with location is to meet in virtual spaces that can be accessed through the Internet. Individuals may participate from anywhere that they can connect.

Curricular variability may present a synchronization problem. Students in different programs may not be studying the same topics at the same time. Teamwork among program developers can help sequence the curricula in such as a way that there are good fits for joint simulated learning experiences.

SUMMARY

Students today are faced with inordinate amounts of information they are expected to learn (Linares, 1999). According to Skiba (2005), current college students, sometimes referred to as the Net Generation or the Millennials, are more hands-on, active learners, multitaskers, and collaborators who embrace technologies as an inherent part of how they communicate and learn. Millennials like to work in teams with peer-to-peer collaboration. All these individuals have different learning styles and require different educational modalities. Meeting those learning needs across the lifespan can be challenging for educators. Simulation in nursing education brings major considerations and challenges, but the benefits appear to outweigh the challenges. In an era when a shortage of nurses in both education and practice is the norm, the goal of increased collaboration may be difficult to achieve. However, if students are to graduate with beginning competency to function in community and interdisciplinary settings, they must participate in meaningful clinical experiences that promote the development of critical thinking and reasoning skills, as well as collaborative learning. Additional research needs to be conducted to evaluate the most effective way to incorporate simulation in collaborative learning experiences.

REFERENCES

Abersold, M., Tschannen, D., Stephens, M., Anderson, P., & Lei, X. (2011). Second Life®: A new strategy in educating nursing students. *Clinical Simulation in Nursing. Advance online publication.* doi:10.1016/j.ecns.2011.05.002.

Agency for Healthcare Research and Quality. (n.d.).*Training guide: Using simulation in TeamSTEPPS training.* In http://www.ahrq.gov/ . Retrieved July 5, 2012 from http://www.ahrq.gov/teamsteppstools /simulation /traininggd.htm.

Anderson, M. , Holmes, T. L., LeFlore, J.L., Nelson, K.A., & Jenkins, T. (2010). *Clinical Simulation in Nursing, 6*(2), e61-e66. doi: 10.1016/j.ecns.2009.08.001.

Booth, T. L., & McMullen-Fix, K. (2012). Innovation CENTER: Collaborative interprofessional simulation in a baccalaureate nursing education program. N*ursing Education Perspectives, 33*(2), 127-129. doi: 10.5480/1536-5026-33.2.127.

Bonnel, W.E., & Vogel Smith, K. (2010). *Teaching technologies in nursing and the health professions: Beyond simulation and online courses.* New York: Springer Publishing Company.

Brewer, E. P. (2011). Successful techniques for using human patient simulation in nursing education. *Journal of Nursing Scholarship, 43*(3), 311-317. doi: 10.1111/j.1547-5069.2011.01405.x.

Chickering, A. W., & Gamson, Z. F. (1987). Seven principles of good practice in undergraduate education. *AAHE Bulletin, 39*(7), 5-10.

Childress, R. M. (2005). An exploration of simulation in nursing education: A collaborative approach utilizing a mock code. *Virginia Nurses Today, 13*(4), 1-3.

Dillon, P. M., Noble, K. A., & Kaplan, L. (2009). Simulation as a means to foster collaborative interdisciplinary education. *Nursing Education Perspectives, 30*(2), 87-90.

Dreifuerst, K. T. (2009). The essentials of debriefing in simulation learning: A concept analysis. *Nursing Education Perspectives, 30*(2), 109–114.

Enlow, M., Shanks, L., Guhde, J., & Perkins, M. (2010). Incorporating interprofessional communication skills (ISBARR) into an undergraduate nursing curriculum. *Nurse Educator, 35*(4), 176-180.

Fink, L. (2009). Teaching in nursing: The faculty role. In D. Billings & J. Halstead (Eds). *Teaching in nursing : A guide for faculty* (3rd ed.) (pp. 3-17), St. Louis, MO: Saunders.

Fountain, R. & Alfred, D. (2009). Student satisfaction with high-fidelity simulation: Does it correlate with learning style? *Nursing Education Perspectives, 30*(2), 96-98.

Freeth, D., Ayida, G., Berridge, E. J., Mackintosh, N., Norris, B., Sadler, C., & Strachan,

A. (2009). Multidisciplinary obstetric simulated emergency scenarios (MOSES): Promoting patient safety in obstetrics with teamwork-focused interprofessional simulations. *Journal of Continuing Education in the Health Professions, 29*(2), 98-104.

Fuhrmann, C., & Zambrana, L. (2010). Speaking the same language: Simulation promotes collaboration among the perinatal team. *Journal of Obstetric, Gynecologic & Neonatal Nursing, 39*, S58.

Gokhale, A.A. (1995). Collaborative learningenhances critical thinking. *Journal of Technology Education,7*(1), 22-30.

Grbach, W., Vincent, L., & Struth, D. (2008). Reformulating SBAR to "I-SBAR-R." Quality and Safety in Nursing Education (QSEN). In *http://www.qsen.org*. Retrieved July 5, 2012 from http://www.qsen.org/teachingstrategy.php?id=33.

Hamilton, S. (Ed.). (1997). *Collaborative learning: Teaching and learning in the arts, sciences, and professional schools* (2nd ed.) (pp. 3-9). Indianapolis, IN: IUPUI Center for Teaching and Learning.

Hamman, W. R. (2004). The complexity of team training: What we have learned from aviation and its applications to medicine. *Quality & Safety in Health Care, 13* (Suppl. 1), 72-79.

Institute of Medicine. (2010).The future of nursing: Leading change, advancing health. In *http://www.iom.edu*. Retrieved July 5, 2012 from http://www.iom.edu/~/media /Files/ Report%20Files/2010/The-Future-ofNursing /Future%20of%20Nursing %202010%20 Recommendations.pdf.

Interprofessional Education Collaborative Expert Panel. (2011). *Core competencies for interprofessional collaborative practice: Report of an expert panel.* Washington, D.C.: Interprofessional Education Collaborative.

Johnson, J. H., Zerwic, J. J., & Theis, S. L. (1999). Clinical simulation laboratory: An adjunct to clinical teaching. *Nurse Educator, 24*(5), 37-41.

Johnson, R. T., & Johnson D. W. (1986). Action research: Cooperative learning in the science classroom. *Science and Children, 24*, 31-32.

The Joint Commission (2008). Hand-off communications: Standardized approach. In *http://www.jointcomission.org*. Retrieved July 5, 2012 from http://www.jointcomission. org/AccreditationAmbulatoryCare/Standards/09_FAQs/NPSG/Communication/ NPSG.02.05.01/.

The Joint Commission (2010). Summary data of sentinel events reviewed by the Joint Commission. In *www.jointcommission.org*. Retrieved July 5, 2012 from http://www. jointcommission.org /assets/1/18/SE_Data_Summary_4Q_2010_(v2).pdf.

CHAPTER 11
INTEGRATING THE QSEN COMPETENCIES INTO SIMULATIONS

Carol F. Durham, EdD, RN, ANEF
Kathryn R. Alden, EdD, MSN, RN, IBCLC

"Every addition to true knowledge is an addition to human power."

—Horace Mann

Quality and safety have always been at the core of nursing. These fundamental concepts continue to evolve as we understand more about what contributes to safe and quality care. The sentinel work of the Institute of Medicine (IOM), where competencies were identified to build a safer health care system, transformed the way the nation as well as health care providers think about patient care and the safety issues surrounding quality care (Kohn, Corrigan, & Donaldson, 2000). In 2007, supported by funding from the Robert Wood Johnson Foundation, Cronenwett and colleagues adapted the work of the IOM to create Quality and Safety Education for Nurses (QSEN) competencies for pre-licensure nursing education. Two years later, graduate-level competencies were published (Cronenwett et al., 2009). The competencies for both levels of nursing education include patient-centered care, teamwork and collaboration, evidence-based practice, quality improvement, safety, and informatics. Knowledge, skills, and attitudes (KSA) exemplars were developed for pre-licensure and graduate nursing education. The graduate KSAs are targeted to a higher level practitioner. (For complete definitions and pre-licensure KSAs for the QSEN competencies, the reader is referred to http://www.QSEN.org/ksas_prelicensure.php. Graduate KSAs can be found at http://www.QSEN.org/ksas_graduate.php.)

The QSEN competencies are intrinsic to nursing education. The knowledge, skills, and attitudes associated with each of the competencies represent core values and concepts that undergird both pre-licensure and graduate nursing curricula. QSEN competencies are inherent to all areas of nursing education — classroom, skills labs, simulation labs, clinical, and post conferences. Across the nation, schools of nursing are adapting curricula to reflect the QSEN competencies. Faculty are creating learning activities that purposefully address the competencies (Durham & Sherwood, 2008).

The use of simulation as an instructional strategy in nursing education provides rich opportunities for educators to emphasize quality and safety (Durham & Alden, 2008, 2012). The widespread use of simulation as an interactive, learner-centered strategy necessarily incorporates the foundational values and concepts that are consistent with program and course objectives. The identification and incorporation of specific QSEN competencies within simulation scenarios should be an intentional and purposeful effort on the part of faculty as they seek to maximize learning experiences for the students and to graduate effective practitioners who enter the work force with the knowledge, skills, and attitudes that promote patient safety and quality care (Durham & Alden, 2012).

This chapter will provide a brief description of the QSEN competencies and will describe methods and examples for intentionally incorporating the QSEN competencies and selected KSAs into pre-, intra-, and post-simulation learning activities.

QUALITY AND SAFETY EDUCATION FOR NURSES COMPETENCIES

The QSEN competencies provide the platform to prepare nurses to "continuously improve the quality and safety of the health care systems in which they work" (Cronenwett et al., 2007, p. 122). Definitions for each of the six competencies are provided in the following paragraphs.

Patient-centered care is defined as care that "recognize[s] the patient or designee as the source of control and full partner in providing compassionate and coordinated care based on respect for patient's preferences, values, and needs" (Cronenwett et al., 2007, p. 123). The focus is on including the patient and/or family as member of the health care team, to individualize the care decisions, clarify expected outcomes, and to empower them to be active participants in the provision of care.

Teamwork and collaboration are defined as "function[ing] effectively within nursing and interprofessional teams, fostering open communication, mutual respect, and shared decision-making to achieve quality patient care" (Cronenwett et al., 2007, p. 125). The focus is on understanding communication styles, utilizing effective strategies for communicating patient data, resolving conflict, and understanding roles, responsibilities, and functions of various team members.

Evidence-based practice is defined as "integrat[ing] best current evidence with clinical expertise and patient/family preferences and values for delivery of optimal health care" (Cronenwett et al., 2007, p. 126). Practitioners are asked to examine the role of evidence in the care of patients, to discriminate between clinical opinion and research, and to articulate sound rationale for deviating from evidence-based practice (Cronenwett et al., 2007).

Quality improvement is defined as "us[ing] data to monitor the outcomes of care processes and us[ing] improvement methods to design and test changes to continuously improve the quality and safety of health care systems" (Cronenwett et al., 2007, p. 127). Quality improvement involves the use of specific processes to measure and improve outcomes of care. Local data is compared with current evidence and prevailing benchmarks; strategies are developed to improve outcomes.

Safety is defined as "minimizing risk of harm to patients and providers through both system effectiveness and individual performance" (Cronenwett et al., 2007, p. 128). The QSEN competency expands the traditional view of safety to consider human factors and design principles, to consider both the benefits and limitations of the technologies to improve safety. Nurses are encouraged to examine causes of error and to consider the impact of national standards on safety outcomes.

Informatics is defined as "us[ing] information and technology to communicate, manage knowledge, mitigate error and support decision-making" (Cronenwett et al., 2007, p. 129). The technology and information management systems are examined in light of patient safety. Informatics integrates the other five competencies, providing improved access to information management and development.

The QSEN competencies and their associated KSAs challenge faculty to re-envision their conceptualization of the familiar concepts found in the competencies. The specificity of the KSAs, stated as measurable objectives, allows faculty to examine the detailed intentions for meeting each competency and to easily incorporate the KSAs into learning objectives for pre- and post-licensure students.

Integrating QSEN Competencies into Simulation

The popularity and widespread use of simulation as an instructional strategy in nursing education implies that educators are utilizing a variety of simulation cases to teach nursing students. Whether faculty are creating original scenarios or utilizing previously developed scenarios or prepackaged ones, it is important to examine the cases to identify where and if the competencies appear. Mapping existing simulation scenarios to the QSEN competencies can be an interactive group activity in which faculty analyze simulation cases to identify the knowledge, skills, and attitudes defined by QSEN. Gaps or omissions in the use of the competencies can be determined and remedied, as desired. Alfes (2010) provides a checklist that can be used by educators to examine existing scenarios for QSEN competencies. It is also useful when designing original scenarios that intentionally incorporate the competencies. Jarzemsky (2009) offers a template for developing scenarios that incorporate the QSEN competencies.

Simulation provides an excellent means for integrating the QSEN competencies into nursing education. Selected QSEN competencies should be deliberately integrated into all simulation scenarios, but it is not necessary for every competency to appear in all simulations. While some of the competencies, such as patient-centered care and safety, are foundational to all simulations, others, such as quality improvement and informatics, must be more intentionally included. For example, many of the KSAs for teamwork and collaboration are key components of each simulated learning experience as students work in nursing and in interprofessional teams. Other KSAs such as authority gradients are not included in every simulation but might be the focus of a simulation used in a leadership and management course.

As faculty create new scenarios based on the desired learning outcomes for specific groups of learners, they can purposefully incorporate concepts and activities centered around the QSEN competencies. Jarzemsky, McCarthy, and Ellis (2010) provide examples of activities that can be placed deliberately in all scenarios, such as requiring students to obtain a verbal order after having reported a change in the patient's status, using a safety scan to detect potential safety hazards, and having all students access patient information from an electronic health record.

Faculty must carefully select the competencies and the associated knowledge, skills, and attitudes that are pertinent to the expected outcomes for the simulated learning experience. The specificity of the KSAs, stated as measurable objectives, allows faculty to examine the detailed intentions for integrating each competency.

At first glance, the comprehensive identification of KSAs for each competency may seem overwhelming to faculty as they attempt to integrate quality and safety competencies into simulation learning activities. Perhaps a novel and somewhat simplistic approach is an appropriate starting point, especially for educators who are unfamiliar with the QSEN work and even more so for those who may be less experienced in creating simulation scenarios. Additionally, for faculty who are experienced with simulation and/or QSEN, a fresh look at integrating the competencies into scenarios can result in heightened effectiveness of simulation as a learner-centered instructional method to emphasize quality and safety. Nursing educators have traditionally divided simulation learning activities into the following three specific phases: pre-simulation, intra-simulation, and post-simulation (debriefing). Similarly, if one considers the language and content of the KSAs, there is a logical parallel with the phases of simulation. Knowledge corresponds with pre-simulation activities, skills with intra-simulation, and attitudes with post-simulation.

The knowledge objectives of the QSEN competencies are cognitive in nature and can be considered foundational to simulation learning activities. Students must have a knowledge base related to the content and purpose of the simulation such that they are able to apply that knowledge in clinical decision-making during the simulation. In constructing a scenario that integrates QSEN competencies, the educator can examine the knowledge objectives for each of the competencies to identify those that are relevant and appropriate. The language of the knowledge objectives includes terms such as describe, examine, explore, differentiate, discriminate, and demonstrate. For example, the competency of patient-centered care includes the knowledge component of "demonstrate comprehensive understanding of the concepts of pain and suffering, including physiologic models of pain and comfort" (Cronenwett et al., 2007, p.123).

The skills objectives of the QSEN competencies can be considered as the active portion of a simulation scenario, or intra-simulation, when learners are engaged in the actual interaction with the patient. This includes the psychomotor skills that are used during the scenario. The terms used by QSEN to describe the skills objectives include action verbs such as assess, provide, elicit, engage, and participate. Skills that correspond with the previously cited knowledge component under patient-centered care include the following:

- Assess presence and extent of pain and suffering

- Assess levels of physical and emotional comfort

- Elicit expectations of patient and family for relief of pain

- Initiate effective treatments to relieve pain and suffering in light of patient values, preferences, and expressed needs (Cronenwett et al., 2007, p. 123).

The QSEN attitudes objective can be directly correlated with post-simulation activities in which debriefing occurs and learners are asked to reflect on their experience, as well as on their knowledge (Alden & Durham, 2012). Terms such as acknowledge, appreciate, value, and respect suggest introspection and the affective nature of reflection as learners consider their simulation experience in relation to previous knowledge, personal and professional experience, emotions, and perceptions. Attitudes that correspond with the previously cited knowledge and skill components under patient-centered care include the following:

- Recognize personally held values and beliefs about the management of pain or suffering

- Appreciate the role of the nurse in relief of all types and sources of pain or suffering

- Recognize that patient expectations influence outcome in management of pain or suffering (Cronenwett et al., 2007, p. 123).

(Note: The authors are aware that many of the KSAs can be targeted to multiple phases of simulation. This would likely be apparent to educators who are experienced with simulation. For ease of understanding, the examples provided will follow the parallel association of the KSAs with the phases of simulation.)

CASE EXAMPLE

To assist educators in understanding how to integrate the QSEN competencies and their associated KSAs into simulation scenarios, the authors provide specific suggestions relative to a case example. This example includes KSAs for pre-licensure students but can also be used as a model for graduate nursing education. See Table 1. The scenario case stem is intended to be used as an example to discuss use of each of the QSEN competencies in simulation.

Table 11-1 Simulation Scenario: Heart Failure
Señora Camilla Gomez is an obese 75-year-old Latina who presented to the emergency department (ED) with shortness of breath, 2+ pitting edema of the extremities, c/o fatigue and weakness, persistent cough, wheezing, lack of appetite, nausea, difficulty concentrating, and palpitations. She has a history of type II diabetes. Her primary language is Spanish, although she speaks some broken English. She is accompanied by her husband, Pablo, who speaks English fluently. Señora Gomez is raising her three school-age grandchildren so that her daughter can work. Both she and her husband are anxious and are uncertain about what to expect. She is anxious to get home to care for her grandchildren and her anxiety is compounded by her concern that her daughter will have to miss work if she is not there to care for the children.

Table 11-2 Patient-Centered Care - *Recognize the patient or designee as the source of control and full partner in providing compassionate and coordinated care based on respect for patient's preferences, values, and needs* (Cronenwett et al., 2007, p.123).

	Pre-simulation	Intra-simulation	Post-Simulation
QSEN KSAs	**K:** *Describe how diverse cultural, ethnic, and social backgrounds function as sources of patient, family, and community values* (Cronenwett et al., 2007, p.123).	**S:** *Elicit patient values, preferences, and expressed needs as part of clinical interview, implementation of care plan, and evaluation of care* (Cronenwett et al., 2007, p.123). **S:** *Communicate patient values, preferences, and expressed needs to other member of health care team* (Cronenwett et al., 2007, p.123). **S:** *Provide patient-centered care with sensitivity and respect for the diversity of human experience* (Cronenwett et al., 2007, p.123).	**A:** *Recognize personally held attitudes about working with patients from different ethnic, cultural, and social backgrounds* (Cronenwett et al., 2007, p.123). **A:** *Willingly support patient-centered care for individuals and groups whose values different from own* (Cronenwett et al., 2007, p.123).
EXEMPLARS	As a pre-simulation assignment, assign one to two evidence -based articles on providing culturally sensitive care to Latino families. Ask students to write a reflective journal entry about how their attitudes and values may differ from the patient for whom they are planning care.	Structure simulation so that there is time for the student to interview the patient about their values and preferences. Create opportunities for the student to communicate the patient values, preferences, and expressed needs to another team member. Include an interpreter in the scenario. Observe how the student communicates with the patient through the interpreter; e.g. does the student face the patient and speak directly to her?	As a component of debriefing, provide opportunities for the care team to discuss their attitudes, sensitivity, and appreciation for the diversity of their patient around the differences and similarities between themselves and the patient and family. Have the students identify strategies they used to support patient-centered care for Señora Gomez and her husband. (Consider access to care for the elderly, Señora Gomez's concern about her responsibilities at home, the language barriers, and the dominance of the male in the Latino culture (husband speaks for wife).

Table 11-3 Teamwork & Collaboration - *Function effectively within nursing and interprofessional teams, fostering open communication, mutual respect, and shared decision-making to achieve quality patient care* (Cronenwett et al., 2007, p.125).

	Pre-simulation	Intra-simulation	Post-Simulation
QSEN KSAs	**K:** *Recognize contributions of other individuals and groups in helping patient/family achieve health goals* (Cronenwett et al., p.125). **K:** *Describe examples of the impact of team functioning on safety and quality of care* (Cronenwett et al., 2007, p.125).	**S:** *Initiate requests for help when appropriate to situation* (Cronenwett et al., 2007, p.125). **S:** *Follow communication practices that minimize risks associated with handoffs among providers and across transitions in care* (Cronenwett et al., 2007, p.125).	**A:** *Respect the centrality of the patient/family as core members of a health care team* (Cronenwett et al., 2007, p.125). **A:** *Respect the unique attributes that members bring to a team, including variation in professional orientations and accountabilities* (Cronenwett et al., 2007, p.125). **A:** *Appreciate the risks associated with handoffs among providers and across transitions in care* (Cronenwett et al., 2007, p.125).
EXEMPLARS	Assign readings about the impact of teamwork and communication on patient safety. In a pre-briefing, discuss relevant mortality and morbidity cases with their root cause being ineffective teamwork, collaboration, and/or communication. Have students reflect on the impact of team functioning on those errors. As a pre-simulation exercise, have students interview various health care providers from their clinical site about their role in patient care.	Embed in the scenario events where the student will need to recognize the need for help, know who to call, and how to elicit help. Build in transitions that require handoffs among providers and across transitions to care such as transfer to the floor from the emergency department and again at discharge home for Señora Gomez.	Elicit from the team how effective they believe they were in making the patient and husband core members of the health care team. Solicit input from the husband about how he perceived the team's inclusion or exclusion of him as a member of the team. Allow the team to reflect on their handoffs — were they effective or not? If taped, view and critique together. Role play exemplars of effective handoffs followed by group feedback.

Table 11-4 **Evidence-Based Practice** – *Integrate best current evidence with clinical expertise and patient/family preferences and values for delivery of optimal health care* (Cronenwett et al., 2007, p.126).

	Pre-simulation	Intra-simulation	Post-Simulation
O S E N K S A s	**K:** *Describe evidence-based practice (EBP) to include the components of research evidence, clinical expertise, and patient/family values* (Cronenwett et al., 2007, p.126).	**S:** *Base individualized care plan on patient values, clinical expertise, and evidence* (Cronenwett et al., 2007, p.126).	**A:** *Value the concept of EBP as integral to determining best clinical practice* (Cronenwett et al., 2007, p.126).
E X E M P L A R S	Assign current evidence-based guidelines for treatment of heart failure. As a group activity, have students construct a table comparing and contrasting best practice for heart failure, chronic obstructive pulmonary disease, and pneumonia. Review the evidence regarding polypharmacy in older adults and the related issues. Are there atypical presentations with the elderly? Have students examine the current evidence about cultural beliefs and practices in the Latino culture as a pre-assignment so that they can adapt them to the individual preferences for Señora Gomez. Provide opportunities for students to learn strategies to express their concern about an order such as using those found in the TeamSTEPPS™ curriculum (TeamSTEPPS, 2008).	Señora Gomez presents with symptoms of heart failure. Her condition worsens as the scenario begins and students must recognize the signs of deterioration in her condition. Embed opportunities for the students to use the evidence that they have reviewed in the pre-simulation assignment in the simulation. For example, when the provider is called, medication orders are given that are contrary to current evidence or do not honor the patient's values. Students are expected to recognize this variance and question the provider's order. Using evidenced-based communication strategies such *I am Concerned*, or *I am Uncomfortable* or *this is a Safety issue* (CUS words) from TeamSTEPPS.	In debriefing, discuss how the evidence influenced the care. Ask if there was evidence that was needed but was not available among the team. Reflect on how best practice is established. Ask students to consider the nursing care they provide in their clinical settings and to discuss where there may not be evidence for what nurses do. If there is no evidence then how is best practice established?

Table 11-5 Quality Improvement – *Use data to monitor the effectiveness of care processes and use improvement methods to design and test changes to continuously improve the quality and safety of health care systems* (Cronenwett et al., 2007, p. 127).

	Pre-simulation	Intra-simulation	Post-Simulation
O S E N K S A s	**K:** *Describe strategies for learning about the outcomes of care in the setting in which one is engaged in clinical practice* (Cronenwett et al., 2007, p.127).	**S:** *Seek information about quality improvement projects in the care setting* (Cronenwett et al., 2007, p.127).	**A:** *Appreciate that continuous quality improvement is an essential part of the daily work of all health professionals* (Cronenwett et al., 2007, p.127).
E X E M P L A R S	Prior to simulation ask students to enter into dialogue with nurse managers in their clinical sites to discuss targeted outcomes. Have students inquire if there are outcomes targeted toward diverse populations, specific disease states such as heart failure, and around certain age groups such as the elderly	During the simulation, have one student observe the processes of care from a quality improvement (QI) perspective. A problem with obtaining needed medication from the pharmacy because it is not available can be a component of the simulation. The observer should recognize this as a system issue and bring it forward for discussion in the debriefing.	Outcomes of care for the Latina women is a topic for discussion in debriefing. Ask reflective questions to allow students to brainstorm ideas for improving some of the issues they have identified through this simulated learning experience, such as how linguistic, cultural, legal, and financial barriers contribute to health care disparities for this group of women.

Table 11-6 Safety – *Minimize risk of harm to patients and providers through both system effectiveness and individual performance* (Cronenwett, et al., 2007, p. 128).

	Pre-simulation	Intra-simulation	Post-Simulation
O S E N K S A s	**K:** *Describe the benefits and limitations of selected safety-enhancing technologies (such as barcodes, Computer Provider Order Entry, medication pumps, and automatic alerts/alarms)* (Cronenwett et al., 2007, p.128).	**S:** *Demonstrate effective use of technology and standardized practices that support safety and quality* (Cronenwett et al., 2007, p.128).	**A:** *Value the contributions of standardization/reliability to safety* (Cronenwett et al., 2007, p.128).
E X E M P L A R S	Review safety principles of medication administration; if students are unfamiliar with IV infusion devices, provide a skills session to teach/review procedures. Review evidence about how safety enhancing technology can be a source of error such as how they contribute to errors such as "alert fatigue" where a nurse ignores the safety alerts.	Students are expected to administer medications using the "six rights" and to follow proper procedures for infusing fluids/medicines via IV pumps. As part of the scenario, have the MD order a new medication that is to be administered as a secondary IV; the student must call the pharmacy and request the medication. When the medication arrives, have students set up the IV with proper tubing, program the pump, and start the IV infusion.	In the debriefing, discuss the procedure that was followed in providing the new medication for the patient; follow the process from MD order to actually administering the IV infusion. Discuss points where errors are most likely to occur and steps to prevent errors. Review the equipment that was used and how to program the IV pump.

Table 11-7 Informatics - *Use information and technology to communicate, manage knowledge, mitigate error, and support decision-making* (Cronenwett, et al., 2007, p. 129).

	Pre-simulation	Intra-simulation	Post-Simulation
O S E N K S A s	**K:** *Identify essential information that must be available in a common database to support patient care* (Cronenwett et al., 2007, p.129).	**S:** *Navigate the electronic medical record* (Cronenwett et al., 2007, p.129).	**A:** *Protect confidentiality of protected health information in electronic health records* (Cronenwett et al., 2007, p.129).
E X E M P L A R S	Assess what students know about health care databases; inquire about specific electronic health record (EHR) systems they have used in their clinical sites. Assess their comfort level in using the systems. Provide readings about EHR and ask student to reflect on how the electronic health record can enhance the care of Señora Gomez. If an EHR is available for the simulation lab and the system is unfamiliar to students, conduct sessions to teach students how to access information and enter data. During the pre-briefing, have students gather data on Señora Gomez from the EHR, such as lab values and EKG.	If using an EHR system for simulation, have students document care; one student may be assigned as recorder and have the responsibility for documenting care provided by the team. Within the simulation it is expected that students not use the husband as a source of medical information. Students should recognize that they need an interpreter.	In debriefing, guide learners in reflective practice about how EHRs enhance safe and quality care. Discuss policies about patient access to medical records and have students debate whether or not patients should have access to their electronic charts. Encourage them to consider ways in which the EHR can contribute to errors. What might be ways to mitigate those errors? Through reflection ask students to appreciate the many ways patient confidentiality can be violated. Do language barriers enhance the likelihood that HIPPA violations might occur? How might nurses protect the protected health information in care provision as well as in the EHR?

SUMMARY

Contemporary nursing education focuses on preparing graduates who are capable of providing safe, quality care that is evidence-based and patient-centered. Teamwork and collaboration, quality improvement, and informatics are essential components of care. Nursing educators can create active learning opportunities through simulation scenarios that intentionally integrate the KSAs of the QSEN competencies. The KSAs parallel the traditional phases of simulation, making it easy for educators to incorporate QSEN competencies into simulation learning activities.

REFERENCES

Alden, K.R., & Durham, C.F. (2012). Integrating reflection in simulation: Structure, content, and processes. In G. Sherwood & S. Horton-Deutsch (Eds.). *Reflective Practice: Transforming Education and Improving Outcomes,* (pp.149-168). Indianapolis, IN: Sigma Theta Tau International.

Cronenwett, L., Sherwood, G., Barnsteiner, J., Disch, J., Johnson, J., Mitchell, P., . . . Warren, J. (2007). Quality and safety education for nurses. *Nursing Outlook, 55*(3), 122-131.

Cronenwett, L., Sherwood, G., Pohl, J., Barnsteiner, J., Moore S., Sullivan, D., . . . Warren, J. (2009). Quality and safety education for advanced nursing practice. *Nursing Outlook, 57*(6), 338-348.

Durham, C. F., & Alden, K. R. (2008). Enhancing patient safety in nursing education through patient simulation. In R. G. Hughes (Ed.), *Patient safety and quality: An evidence-based handbook for nurses* (pp. 3.221 – 3.260). Rockville, MD: Agency for Healthcare Research and Quality.

Durham, C. F., & Sherwood, G. (2008). Educational approaches to bridge the quality gap. *Journal of Urologic Nursing, 28*, 431-438.

Jarzemsky, P. (2009). A template for simulation scenario development that incorporates QSEN competencies. In *www.qsen.org*. Retrieved July 6, 2012 from http://www.qsen.org / teachingstrategy.php?id=70

Jarzemsky, P., McCarthy, J., & Ellis, N. (2010). Incorporating quality and safety education for nurses competencies in simulation scenario design. *Nurse Educator, 35*(2), 90-92.

Kohn, L. T., Corringan, J. M. & Donaldson, M. S. (Eds). (2000). *To err is human: Building a safer health system*. Institute of Medicine (IOM), Washington, DC: National Academy Press.

CHAPTER 12
SUMMARY AND FUTURE CONSIDERATIONS

Mary Anne Rizzolo, EdD, RN, FAAN, ANEF

"The important thing is not to stop questioning.

Curiosity has its own reason for existing."

–Albert Einstein

Simulation in some form has probably been used as a teaching strategy in nursing education since the first nurse tried to teach the first nursing student how to do a task properly. As our understanding of teaching and learning progressed, so did the simulations that were used. Everyone who is reading this book can recall some experiences in the nursing school lab regulating an IV drip, practicing blood pressure measurement on a fellow student, or perhaps positioning "Mrs. Chase," a manikin developed in 1910 (Herrmann, 2008). As audio/visual materials, then computers, were incorporated into the lab, slides, videos, and computer-assisted instruction programs were used to demonstrate skills prior to practice. These multifaceted experiences incorporating media, instruction by faculty, practice, and return demonstrations increased the amount of time that students spent in the lab.

Some innovative educators used the nursing lab in more creative ways, developing, for example, an experience in which the manikin was an unconscious fresh post-op patient, and challenging students to do a quick assessment and discover such things as a name mismatch between the patient's armband and the chart, or "bleeding" from the abdominal incision, which could be seen only by the thorough student who turned the patient to his/her side. But, in general, most labs were used to practice skills.

Large learning resource centers began to appear in the late 1970s, when enterprising faculty in some schools secured funds from grants and other sources to build expansive centers containing equipment that was as good as or better than that which is found in most hospitals. Some purchased cameras to record student practice sessions, others had large audiovisual production capabilities, and still others used their funding to hire and train standardized patients, who described their health care problems and allowed students to practice physical examination and interviewing skills. But the advent of computerized manikins and task trainers and the decrease in the cost of that equipment has brought us to a new era in the development and use of all kinds of simulations. The first edition of this book, the first of its kind for nurse educators, was the work of an innovative, creative group of nurse educators who wished to share what they learned during the course of a three-year, multi-site project that tested simulation models and contributed to the refinement of the body of knowledge related to the use of simulation in nursing education. The second edition has some new authors, new chapters, and new content, but it retains its focus as a basic, foundational book for those who are just beginning their simulation journey or for those who wish to validate their simulation practice by reading what experts in the field have learned about designing, implementing, and evaluating scenarios.

Chapter 1. Using Simulation in Nursing Education provides a brief history on the use of simulations and the evolution of nursing as a practice-based discipline, one that is ideal for incorporating simulation as a teaching-learning activity. A broad definition of simulation is presented, and the increased use of simulation in nursing education since the original edition of this book was printed is documented. A variety of evidence-based articles are cited that have documented simulation's effectiveness. The advantages and challenges of developing simulations and incorporating them into the curriculum are discussed, along with an appeal for recognition of the need for faculty development in the use of simulation and research that focuses on effectiveness and transferability to patient care.

Chapter 2. Simulations: Education and Ethics has been updated to include recent efforts to promote interprofessional education and practice to provide a safer environment for patients. The argument that simulation provides an excellent teaching and evaluation environment for students, but nurse educators should consider whether or not they have an ethical responsibility to provide simulated experiences to insure patient safety is proposed through a list of thoughtful but challenging questions. The principles of justice, autonomy, beneficence, nonmaleficence, veracity, and compassion are discussed to argue for student experiences using simulations prior to clinical practice. Educators are reminded that they need to advocate for the interests of patients as well as students, and a change in the culture of nursing education and moving toward more use of simulation can facilitate that movement.

Chapter 3. Theoretical Framework for Simulation Design contains updates to the NLN/Jeffries Simulation Framework. The framework, originally developed for the NLN/Laerdal Simulation Study (see Appendix A) is described, including the various learning theories that were considered in the early stages of conceptualization. The advantages of using a framework that specifies relevant variables and their relationships to guide the design, implementation, and evaluation of simulations, and to conduct systematized research are delineated. Changes in the framework are based on the work of a research task force convened by the International Nursing Association for Clinical Simulation and Learning that proposed changing the names of two components — "teacher" to "facilitator" and "student" to "participant." Recent evidence-based articles that support each component have been added and several areas for future research are proposed.

Chapter 4. Designing Simulation Scenarios to Promote Learning has several new authors and almost all of the content is different from the 2007 version. It begins by discussing how to decide what simulations to write. The authors compare writing a scenario to writing a story or play, and provide suggestions on how to approach the beginning, middle, and ending when writing the story. In each writing phase they discuss pitfalls and how to avoid them. Peer review to establish validity and piloting with a targeted population of learners is strongly encouraged. The value of having a template to provide consistency and to insure that no essential elements are overlooked is recommended.

Chapter 5. Curriculum Integration of Clinical Simulation is a new chapter that replaces the chapter titled "Practical Suggestions for Implementing Simulations" in the original edition of the book. It describes a systematic approach for tackling the task of integrating simulation throughout the nursing curriculum. A seven-step plan includes forming a team composed of those who will be essential for success, the process for curriculum review, identification of resources and development of policies, along with an implementation and evaluation plan.

Chapter 6. Integrating Guided Reflection into Simulated Learning Experiences provides an overview of the concept of reflecting, beginning with its philosophic underpinnings. The two types of reflection described by Schön, reflection–in-action and reflection-on-action, are expanded to include reflection-beyond-action. Several new articles that support the importance of guided reflection in nursing are cited to support the original work of experts in nursing education who have written about the development of clinical judgment and reasoning, and the relationship of reflective thinking to this process. The tables on establishing a safe environment for reflection and research questions that need to be addressed when integrating reflection into simulation have been expanded.

Chapter 7. Debriefing: an Essential Component for Learning in Simulation Pedagogy presents a comprehensive overview of debriefing, complete with supporting research. The authors emphasize that debriefing is an essential component of all types of simulation experiences from manikin- and screen-based through standardized patients and serious gaming. It addresses practical issues, such as the length of a debrief session and when and where it should occur, and more complex issues, like the faculty role during debriefing and how to modify the debriefing process to meet the needs of learners. Four commonly used debriefing methods are described and a special section on strategies to guide reflection includes a table that provides suggested open-ended questions to encourage reflection-on-action. Two tools for evaluating debriefing are described. The chapter concludes with suggestions on how to deal with special debriefing circumstances, like those involving large groups or interprofessional teams, and how to debrief when there has been poor performance.

Chapter 8. Evaluation: A Critical Step in Simulation Practice and Research provides an overview of basic concepts about evaluation and explicates them with examples from recent research studies. The authors begin by explaining each step in the process of systematic evaluation — identifying the purpose of the evaluation, determining a timeframe, developing the plan, selecting appropriate instruments, collecting data, and interpreting data. The many types of evaluation and the various points when evaluation is useful are presented, from evaluating the simulation design to high-level studies that endeavor to link simulation to improved patient outcomes. A summary of selected types of evaluation instruments is provided, along with examples of some that were developed for the first NLN study (Jeffries & Rizzolo, 2007) and have been used extensively since then. The types of reliability and validity and strategies for obtaining evidence about these measures are also explained. While it is gratifying to note that the reference list at the end of the chapter has more than doubled from this chapter's previous version, much more evaluation and research is needed to discover and inform the effective use of simulation.

Chapter 9. Setting Up a Simulation Center discusses the fact that a clinical simulation center is intended to replicate a "real world" clinical setting or situation as closely as possible to provide learning experiences that allow learners to integrate theory and practice, develop clinical judgment, and ensure patient safety. There are a myriad of decisions that need to be made when designing and building a new center or renovating existing space. This chapter approaches those challenges by focusing not only on the physical environment, but also on its function, including collaboration, governance, organization, personnel, technology, space, supplies, resources, and equipment. The authors include everything from establishing a design team and governance structure to administrative concerns such as funding sources, budgetary, and personnel issues to very practical matters such as janitorial services, parking, and hints for finding sources of free supplies. Valuable advice is provided on floor plans, and purchase and maintenance of equipment, hardware and software, along with guidance on day-to-day operations, scheduling, inventory, and restocking management.

Chapter 10. Using Collaboration to Enhance the Effectiveness of Simulated Learning in Nursing Education. Today's complex health care environment requires collaboration and communication among the health care team to ensure safe patient care. Simulation in health care education is an effective way to facilitate this collaboration. Additions to this chapter focus on communication and include reports of sentinel events and the recommendations of the Joint Commission and the Agency for Healthcare Research and Quality related to standardized communication to improve patient safety. The TeamsSTEPPS and SBAR/ISBARR tools are cited. Examples of various types of collaborative learning experiences are described, including student-to-student, faculty-to-student, academic faculty-to-clinicians, and interdisciplinary exercises. The variety of roles that faculty can play when a simulation is designed to promote collaboration are discussed. Future trends for interprofessional education and the possibilities for simulation in virtual environments are discussed. The European Union's initiative to fund the standardization of virtual patient design and implementation is mentioned as a way to surmount some barriers to using simulation in virtual worlds.

Chapter 11. Integrating the QSEN Competencies into Simulations begins with background on the Quality and Safety Education for Nurses (QSEN) initiative, followed by descriptions and definitions for each competency — patient-centered care, teamwork and collaboration, evidence-based practice, quality improvement, safety, and informatics. Methods for intentionally incorporating the competencies with their associated knowledge, skills, and attitudes (KSAs) are discussed. A short case study is provided, followed by specific examples on how to integrate the KSAs for each competency into the three phases of simulation — pre-simulation, intra-simulation, and post-simulation or debriefing.

CONCLUDING THOUGHTS

The chapters in this book have presented many advantages for using simulations in the education of tomorrow's nurses. Some of the most compelling reasons include

- Providing a safe, risk-free environment where students can practice without the fear of harming a client.

- Supplying every student with an opportunity to rehearse low-frequency, high-risk clinical experiences that they would otherwise never experience.

- Ensuring that every student has the knowledge and skills to care for patients with commonly occurring health care problems.

- Practicing collaboration, leadership, and delegation skills with other health care providers

- Allowing students to safely experience and work through feelings around sensitive, uncomfortable, and controversial situations they may encounter in practice (e.g., abortion, addicted or abused clients, and clients or families who are dealing with end-of-life issues).

When students are immersed in a scenario where they must use all their skills to assess a patient, then formulate and implement a plan of care, they become aware of the gaps in their knowledge — a sobering experience and a powerful motivator for learning.

Another advantage became evident to me recently when a student told me that in simulation he could see how his many fellow students approach their patients and provide nursing care and that encouraged him to consider different ways to think about his own practice of nursing. And of course, we cannot forget how simulation reveals the strengths and weaknesses of a curriculum. Many faculty relay the experience of watching their students in a simulation and being surprised — either positively or negatively — by what they see. "But we taught them how to do ____. How could they forget?" is a commonly heard comment.

It is encouraging to see how much simulation has evolved since the first edition of this book was released in 2007. The reference lists at the end of each chapter have grown significantly, conferences and workshops on simulation have proliferated, and national initiatives have emerged. The National League for Nursing's Simulation Innovation Resource Center (http://sirc.nln.org) was launched and now has 16 online courses and many other resources to assist faculty. The International Association for Clinical Simulation and Learning (2011) released a set of guidelines and is beginning to work on more. This organization is also examining the NLN/Jeffries Simulation Framework to determine its readiness to move to a theory. The Society for Simulation in Healthcare (http://www.ssih.org) launched an accreditation of simulation centers program and will offer the first certification for health care simulation educators this summer. The results of the National Council of State Boards of Nursing Study (2012) currently underway will tell us the amount of clinical practice that can be replaced by simulation. The NLN's Project to Explore the Use of Simulation for High Stakes Assessment (2010) will inform what needs to be done to develop and implement simulations for summative assessment.

While much research has been done in the last five years, much more is needed — to answer relatively simple questions, such as how much time is appropriate for a specific simulation or for a specific level of student, and to explore the more complex questions, such as whether the use of simulations throughout the curriculum leads to better critical thinking and clinical judgment skills in graduates. Researchers also should explore whether a simulated experience prior to clinical practice leads to less anxiety and more learning during clinical experiences with patients. The rich qualitative data that surfaces when students tell faculty about their experiences with simulation continues to generate more complex research questions.

Any type of research on educational strategies and practice is difficult. There are many challenges, and it is impossible to control some variables such as past experiences of students. Our evaluation instruments are limited, but we are beginning to see new tools being developed (Kardong-Edgren, Adamson, & Fitzgerald, 2010). We must advance the science of nursing education to confront these challenges and inform our teaching practice.

Today's students have grown up with technology. They expect and deserve active, student-centered teaching and learning that incorporates the latest technological advancements to help them learn efficiently, effectively, and safely so they can provide quality care to patients. And technology is advancing at an increasingly rapid pace. Consider how quickly we have progressed from the simple, computer-assisted instruction programs of the 1980s to virtual hospitals and complex patient situations with multiple paths and branches. In the last edition, I wrote, "The manikins of today will be wireless tomorrow," and that has already happened! Our next generation of manikins will walk as well as talk, and they will simulate sophisticated symptoms like changes in skin texture and sensation. Soon we will be able to immerse our students in a virtual health care environment, complete with entire units filled with patients and other health care personnel, complete with all of the sights, sounds, and smells unique to that environment. Will faculty be prepared to harness and shape the learning environments of tomorrow and create meaningful learning, evidence-based experiences for their students? We hope this book can provide a beginning pathway to help faculty work toward that goal.

References

Herrmann, E.K. (2008). Remembering Mrs. Chase. Imprint, 55(2), 52-55. International Nursing Association for Clinical Simulation and Learning Board of Directors (2011, August). Standards of best practice: Simulation. *Clinical Simulation in Nursing, 7*(4S), s10-s11. doi:10.1016/j.ecns.2011.05.007

Jeffries, P.R. & Rizzolo, M.A. (2007) *Designing and implementing models for the innovative use of simulation to teach nursing care of ill adults and children: A national, multi-site, multi-method study.* Retrieved April 18, 2012 from http://www.nln.org/research/LaerdalReport.pdf.

Kardong-Edgren, S., Adamson, K., & Fitzgerald, C. (2010). A review of currently published evaluation instruments for human patient simulation. *Clinical Simulation in Nursing, 6*(1), e25-e35. doi: 10.1016/jecns.2009.08.004.

National Council of State Boards of Nursing (2012). *NCSBN national simulation study.* Retrieved April 18, 2012 from https://www.ncsbn.org/2094.htm.

National League for Nursing (2010) *National League for Nursing task group tackles high stakes testing.* Retrieved April 18, 2012 from http://www.nln.org/newsreleases / highstakes_testing_ 061110.htm.

APPENDIX A
AUTHOR PROFILES

Pamela R. Jeffries, PhD, RN, FAAN, ANEF

Professor, Associate Dean of Academic Affairs, Johns Hopkins University School of Nursing, Baltimore, MD

Dr. Pamela R. Jeffries is the associate dean of academic affairs at Johns Hopkins School of Nursing. She has over 25 years of teaching experience in the classroom, learning laboratory, and clinical setting with undergraduate nursing students. Dr. Jeffries has been awarded several teaching awards including the National League for Nursing Lucile Petry Leone Award for nursing education, the prestigious Elizabeth Russell Belford Award for teaching excellence given by Sigma Theta Tau, and numerous outstanding faculty awards presented by the graduating nursing classes.

Dr. Jeffries was named project director of the three-year National League for Nursing (NLN/Laerdal) Simulation Study. She worked with eight project coordinators selected by the NLN from over 150 applicants. The overarching purpose of the exploratory, national, multi-site project was to study various parameters related to the use of simulation in basic nursing education programs and selected student outcomes. She also served as the project director for a second NLN/Laerdal grant focused on faculty development for designing and implementing simulations. Nine web-based courses have been designed and marketed for this project in addition to a global simulation website called the "Simulation Innovation Resource Center" (SIRC) that contains many resources for simulation educators.

Dr. Jeffries has been involved with numerous technological development projects, including a Small Business Innovative Resource (SBIR) grant developing a CD ROM on clinical skills in nursing, a Small Business Technology Transfer STTR grant that consisted of developing an online acute care respiratory module for nurse practitioners, and was co-primary investigator (PI) on a federally-funded Department of Education Grant (Funding from Post-Secondary Education- FIPSE) to develop three online critical care courses. Most recently she is serving as PI on an American Heart Association grant to study Advanced Cardiac Life Support (ACLS) instruction using high-fidelity manikins and is co-director on a five-year Health Resources and Services Administration (HRSA) grant that is directed toward faculty development to teach nurse educators about emerging technologies. Her research and scholarship of teaching are focused on studying learning outcomes, instructional design, new pedagogies, innovative teaching strategies, interprofessional education, and delivery of content using technology and simulated learning.

KATIE ANNE ADAMSON, PhD, RN

Assistant Professor, University of Washington, Tacoma, WA

Dr. Katie Anne Adamson is an Assistant Professor at the University of Washington – Tacoma, where she teaches in the nursing and healthcare leadership programs. Her research areas include human patient simulation, nursing education, evaluation, instrument development, and psychometrics. When she is not teaching and doing research, Dr. Adamson enjoys hiking, biking, swimming, and traveling.

KATHRYN R. ALDEN, EdD, MSN, RN, IBCLC

Clinical Associate Professor, University of North Carolina- Chapel Hill, Apex, NC

Dr. Kathryn R. Alden is an experienced nurse and educator, having taught in the undergraduate nursing program at the University of North Carolina – Chapel Hill for 25 years. She was an early adopter of high-fidelity simulation and has developed numerous cases for maternal and newborn nursing. Dr. Alden has authored simulation scenarios for Elsevier's Simulation Learning System and has co-authored chapters on simulation and patient safety for nationally recognized texts. She is the co-editor of Mosby's Maternity and Women's Health Care (10th ed.) and associate editor for Maternity Nursing (8th ed.).

DIANE S. ASCHENBRENNER, MS, APRN, RN, BC

Instructor, Undergraduate Course Coordinator, Faculty Coordinator, the Simulation and Nursing Practice Labs, Johns Hopkins University School of Nursing, Baltimore, MD

Diane S. Aschenbrenner is an instructor and faculty coordinator for the Simulation and Nursing Practice Labs at the Johns Hopkins School of Nursing. She established and is now the Faculty Coordinator for the Simulation and Nursing Practice Labs. In this role she is responsible for integrating simulation into the School of Nursing's undergraduate and graduate curriculum. Numerous national and international nursing educators have visited and consulted with her at the Johns Hopkins University Simulation and Nursing Practice Labs. Her areas of scholarly expertise and interest include clinical simulations; teaching strategies; pharmacology; medication administration techniques and preventing errors; medical-surgical nursing, adults; and teaching clinical skills. She has presented at 18 international and 35 domestic conference presentations related to simulation, teaching strategies, and skills acquisition. She has provided international consulting related to teaching nursing skills (Egypt, 2006), nursing documentation (China, 2008), and simulation (Switzerland, 2012).

She is the lead author of Aschenbrenner and Venable's *Drug Therapy in Nursing*, a pharmacology text for nursing students currently in its fourth edition. She is, since 2003, a monthly columnist and contributing editor for the American Journal of Nursing where her Drug Watch column is a widely read feature. She was a coauthor of the chapter "Clinical Reasoning and Judgment" in the third edition of Frith & Clark's book Distance Education in Nursing.

MARY L. CATO MSN, RN

Assistant Professor of Nursing, Simulation and Clinical Learning Center, Oregon Health & Science University School of Nursing, Portland, OR

Mary Cato has been teaching with simulation for over eight years and has facilitated the integration of simulation into the OHSU nursing curriculum. She was one of the NLN SIRC authors and has contributed to three of the SIRC courses. Ms. Cato has also been a part of the NLN Advancing Care Excellence for Seniors project, and has authored one of the unfolding case studies, which includes three progressive simulation cases. She continues to teach in all levels of the OHSU undergraduate nursing programs, and co-teaches a graduate course on simulation in nursing education. Ms. Cato is currently engaged in simulation research as part of her doctoral studies.

PAUL M. COLLINS, CCEMT-P

Simulation Coordinator, Indiana University, Indianapolis, IN

Paul Collins is the simulation coordinator for the Simulation Center at Fairbanks Hall. He is originally from Grand Rapids, Michigan, where he worked as a medical educator for seven years. He moved to Indianapolis to work at the Indiana School of Nursing as their simulation coordinator in 2008 and became the simulation coordinator for the Simulation Center at Fairbanks Hall in August 2009.

SHARON I. DECKER, PhD, RN, ANEF, FAAN

Professor, Covenant Health System Endowed Chair in Simulation and Nursing Education, Anita Thigpen Perry School of Nursing, Texas Tech University Health Sciences Center, Lubbock, TX

Dr. Sharon Decker is a professor and the Covenant Health System Endowed Chair in Simulation and Nursing Education at the Anita Thigpen Perry School of Nursing at the Texas Tech University Health Sciences Center (TTUHSC) in Lubbock. She is the director of the F. Marie Hall SimLife Center and the director of the Health Sciences Center's Quality Enhancement Program (QEP): Interprofessional Team. As a member of international, interprofessional simulation organizations, Dr. Decker has promoted the development of the science and pedagogy of simulation. Dr. Decker's scholarship focuses on the pedagogy of simulation. Her educational research, supported by multiple grants, is related to how simulation can be used to improve learning and promote professional competencies. She presents nationally and internationally on topics related to simulation and interprofessional teamwork and serves as a national and international consultant to assist nurse educators in the integration of simulation into curricula and competency assessments. Dr. Decker received her BSN from Baylor University, her MSN for the University of Texas at Arlington, and her PhD from Texas Woman's University. She is a fellow in the National League for Nursing's Academy of Nursing Education and a fellow in the American Academy of Nursing.

KRISTINA THOMAS DREIFUERST, PhD, RN, ACNS-BC, CNE

Assistant Professor, Indiana University School of Nursing, Indianapolis, IN

Dr. Kristina Thomas Dreifuerst is an assistant professor at Indiana University School of Nursing in Indianapolis, Indiana. Dr. Dreifuerst received her BA in nursing from Luther College, Decorah, Iowa, and her MS in nursing from the University of Wisconsin – Madison. Dr. Dreifuerst has taught undergraduate and graduate nurses for many years in Wisconsin and Michigan and she currently teaches graduate students in the nurse educator major at IU. She is a 2011 NLN-Jonas Scholar for Excellence in Nursing Education Research. Her program of research focuses on the development of clinical reasoning in prelicensure nurses. Dr. Dreifuerst is the author of the Debriefing for Meaningful Learning method of clinical and simulation debriefing.

CAROL F. DURHAM, EdD, RN, ANEF

Clinical Professor and the Director of the Education-Innovation-Simulation Learning Environment, University of North Carolina School of Nursing, Chapel Hill, NC

Dr. Durham is a clinical professor and the director of the Education-Innovation-Simulation Learning Environment at the University of North Carolina at Chapel Hill School of Nursing. She has developed many simulated learning experiences for a variety of learners including undergraduate students, nurse practitioner students, interprofessional students in nursing, medicine and pharmacy, as well as practicing registered nurse, licensed practical nurses and nursing assistants. She has been instrumental in integrating simulation into the undergraduate curriculum and select courses in the graduate program. Dr. Durham is a QSEN faculty, assisting nurse educators to integrate Quality Safety Education for Nurses (QSEN) into simulation within their curriculum. Dr. Durham is a fellow of the Academy of Nursing Education and faculty for the National League of Nursing Simulation Innovation Resource Center (SIRC). She is on the editorial review board for the Clinical Simulation in Nursing Journal. Dr. Durham has consulted with nursing schools around the nation providing faculty development around simulation, quality, and safety.

SCOTT A. ENGUM, MD

Professor of Surgery, Indiana University School of Medicine; Director, the Simulation Center at Fairbanks Hall, Indiana University of Health, Indianapolis, IN

Dr. Scott A. Engum completed his general surgery residency training in 1994 and his pediatric surgery fellowship training in 1996. He is a professor of surgery and attending faculty member at the James Whitcomb Riley Hospital for Children, where he instructs medical students, surgery residents, and pediatric surgery fellows. Dr. Engum served on the planning/design and operational groups for the interprofessional simulation center build-out that was completed on the Indiana University Health/IUPUI campus in 2009 and serves as the director of the center.

CHERYL FEKEN, MS, RN

Assistant Professor of Nursing, Clinical Simulation Coordinator, Tulsa Community College, Tulsa, OK

Cheryl Feken is the clinical simulation coordinator at Tulsa Community College. She was a reviewer for the NLN Laerdal SimMan Scenarios, Volumes I and II and VitalSim Scenarios. Ms. Feken co-authored a chapter with Dr. Sharon Decker and Dr. Teresa Gore in Essential of e-Learning for Nurse Educators. Ms. Feken has been on the board of International Nursing Association of Clinical Simulation Learning (INACSL) for three years and participated in development of "Standards of Best Practices: Simulation" published August 2011 in Clinical Simulation in Nursing. Ms. Feken has been active in the Oklahoma Healthcare Workforce Center, promoting simulation as an education resource. She has presented at several conferences on topics such as scenario development, implementation, and budgeting.

JULIE MCAFOOES, MS, RN-BC, CNE, ANEF

Web Development Manager, Chamberlain College of Nursing, Downers Grove, IL

Julie McAfooes is a web development manager for the Chamberlain College of Nursing where she collaborates with faculty and developers to design and maintain online courses in undergraduate and graduate programs. Her research interest is simulation, in particular virtual simulation, which was the focus of a research study on Second Life when she was a HITS scholar. Ms. McAfooes has served as an instructional designer for the NLN Simulation Innovation Resource Center (SIRC). She is the project manager of the NLN/Jeffries Simulation Framework effort to advance the framework to a theory. She is board certified by American Nursing Credential Center (ANCC) in nursing professional development, and certified as a nurse educator (CNE) by the NLN. As the former nurse educator for FITNE, Inc., she gave more than 200 presentations promoting the use of technology in nursing education.

LESLEY BRAUN MILGROM, MSN, RN, CNE

Clinical Assistant Professor, Indiana University, Indianapolis, IN

Lesley Milgrom is a clinical assistant professor at Indiana University teaching in the undergraduate baccalaureate of science in nursing program. She received a bachelor of art in nursing from Simmons College, Boston, and Master of Science in nursing from Indiana University, Indianapolis. Her clinical background and area of teaching is in critical care and medical-surgical nursing. She is the undergraduate liaison for simulation at Indiana University School of Nursing. She has developed and implemented simulations in the undergraduate nursing program and coordinates the annual SIM Institute at Indiana University. She has reviewed and designed simulations for Laerdal. She is actively involved with the integrations of interprofessional education into the curriculum and her research focus is interprofessional communication and simulation.

REBA MOYER CHILDRESS, MSN, RN, FNP, FAANP, ANEF

Assistant Professor of Nursing and Clinical Simulation Learning Center Coordinator, University of Virginia School of Nursing, Charlottesville, VA

Reba Moyer Childress is a passionate advocate for simulation in health care education and has presented at a variety of conferences nationally and internationally to promote the use of simulation in education and practice. In 2006, she founded the Virginia State Simulation Alliance (VASSA), Inc. As the director, Ms. Childress and her role in VASSA were instrumental in obtaining approval from the Virginia Board of Nursing to accept simulation as direct clinical hours in the state of Virginia. Ms. Childress also is a founding member of the International Nursing Association for Clinical Simulation and Learning (INACSL) and was recognized for her contributions to INACSL with their service award in 2006.

PATRICIA RAVERT, PhD, RN, CNE, ANEF, FAAN

Associate Dean for Undergraduate Studies and the Nursing Learning Center and Clinical Simulation Laboratory Coordinator, Brigham Young University College of Nursing, Provo, Utah

Dr. Patricia Ravert is the associate dean for undergraduate studies and the Nursing Learning Center and Clinical Simulation Laboratory coordinator in the College of Nursing at Brigham Young University, Provo, Utah. Dr. Ravert has been using high-fidelity simulation since 2001 and has facilitated many simulation sessions. Her work has also involved integrating high-fidelity simulation sessions across the baccalaureate curriculum. She was one of the experts on the NLN/Laerdal Simulation Innovation Resource Center project and authored or co-authored two of the courses. Dr. Ravert served as the BSN representative on the board of directors for the International Association of Clinical Simulation and Learning (INACSL) and currently serves as the research advisor.

KRISTEN J. ROGERS, MSN, RN

Service Excellence Director, Washington Hospital School of Nursing, Washington, PA

Kristen Rogers has been a part of the nursing profession for 24 years, with 15 years focused on nursing education. In her present position as service excellence director, she collaborates with health care team members to enhance the patient and family experience. In her previous position as assistant director of the school of nursing, she conducted ongoing evaluation of the curriculum and facilitated program evaluation n accordance with National League for Nursing Accrediting Commissions (NLNAC) standards and criteria and the State Board of Nursing standards. She served on the NLN Task Group on Clinical Nursing Education and the NLN Education Technology and Information Management Advisory Council. Her publications include co-authoring one chapter in Clinical Nursing Education: Current Reflections, headlines from the NLN in Nursing Education Perspectives, and co-authoring two chapters in Simulation in Nursing Education: From Conceptualization to Evaluation (1st edition). She has also been a presenter at national conferences.

MARY ANNE RIZZOLO, EdD, RN, FAAN, ANEF

Senior Director for Professional Development, National League for Nursing, New York, NY

Dr. Mary Anne Rizzolo is responsible for the professional development programs offered by the NLN, served as the staff liaison to the NLN/Laerdal Simulation Study, and staffs NLN's Educational Technology and Information Management Advisory Council and its three task groups: Informatics Competencies, Information Management and the Educational Process, and Instructional Technologies. She previously developed educational software products for nursing education, and was the principal investigator of a special projects grant from the Division of Nursing that developed one of the first nursing websites, AJN Online, which evolved into the current NursingCenter.com.

JULIE SETTLES MSN, ACNP-BC, CEN

Co-Program Coordinator of the Acute Care Nurse Practitioner (NP) Program, Indiana University, Indianapolis, IN

Julie Settles is the co-program coordinator of the Acute Care NP program at Indiana University. She has worked as an NP in the cardiovascular critical care unit and currently practices as an NP in the emergency department. She has worked as a tactical medic for the FBI SWAT team. Ms. Settles has been designing and implementing simulations for both undergraduate and graduate program for several years. She was a reviewer for the Laerdal NLN nursing scenarios I and was the content expert and developer for the Laerdal NLN scenarios volume II. She has been involved in the review of Sim Man 3 G software and her recent work includes SimJr. and SimMom. Julie lectures nationally and internationally on simulation theory, design and implementation and is co-project investigator on four simulation-based research projects, including an American Heart Association sponsored project and a large multi-site study using Harvey the Cardiac patient simulator, sponsored by the Gordon Center for Medical Education. She is in her doctoral program at Rush University and is studying the use of high-fidelity human simulators to increase self-efficacy and reduce cognitive errors at the bedside.

BRUCE R. WILLIAMS, RN, MS, MSN, EMT

Simulation Technician, Indiana University of Health, Simulation Center at Fairbanks Hall, Indianapolis, IN

Bruce R. Williams received his associate's degree in nursing from Vincennes University (1994) and bachelor's degree in nursing from University of Southern Indiana (2000). He completed a master's degree in occupational safety management while attending Indiana State University (2002) then completed a master's degree in nursing from University of Southern Indiana (2008). He began his clinical career in the intensive care unit at Welborn Baptist Hospital in Evansville, Indiana. From the ICU he transferred to the emergency department and then flight nursing in Evansville and Lexington, Kentucky. Other areas of clinical experience include industrial medicine and organ procurement. In 2005, Mr. Williams became nursing faculty for the Ivy Tech Community College of Indiana, Southwest Campus. He moved to Indianapolis in May 2011 to work at the Simulation Center at Fairbanks Hall.

APPENDIX B
FINAL REPORT OF THE NLN/LAERDAL SIMULATION STUDY

Project Title

Designing and Implementing Models for the Innovative Use of Simulation to Teach Nursing Care of Ill Adults and Children: A National, Multi-Site, Multi-Method Study

Project Sponsors

National League for Nursing and Laerdal Medical

Report Prepared by

Pamela R. Jeffries, PhD, RN, FAAN, Project Director
Associate Professor and Associate Dean for Undergraduate Programs
Indiana University School of Nursing

Mary Anne Rizzolo, EdD, RN, FAAN
Senior Director for Professional Development
National League for Nursing

Project Period

June 1, 2003 to May 31, 2006
Copyright © 2006 by the National League for Nursing
61 Broadway, 33rd Floor
New York, NY 10006

PURPOSES OF THE PROJECT

The purposes of this national, multi-site, multi-method project were fourfold, as follows:

1) To develop and test models that nursing faculty can implement when using simulation to promote student learning,

2) To develop a cadre of nursing faculty who can use simulation in innovative ways to enhance student learning,

3) To contribute to the refinement of the body of knowledge related to the use of simulation in nursing education, and

4) To demonstrate the value of collaboration between the corporate and not-for-profit worlds.

Goals of the Research

The research goals were to explore how to design simulations, implement simulations as a teaching strategy, and evaluate selected learning outcomes using simulations. Specifically, the study was designed to do the following:

1) Develop a teaching-learning framework incorporating simulations that nurse educators can use to help guide the development, implementation, and evaluation of the use of simulations in nursing education.

2) Describe and test a design that is theoretically based and can be used to develop nursing simulations that promote good learning outcomes.

3) Explore relationships among the theoretical concepts of the simulation framework to assess the existence and importance of these concepts.

4) Test and analyze selected outcomes when implementing a nursing simulation based on the proposed theoretical concepts using an experimental design.

Project Phases

Phase I: June 2003 to December 2003

The aim of this phase was to organize the eight project coordinators and one projectdirector to discuss the project and set specific directions for the study. Specifically, Phase I was designed to clarify the purpose of the study; discuss the nature of participating in a national, multi-site study; conduct a review of the simulation literature; apply for Internal Review Board (IRB) approval at each institution to conduct the research study there; develop a research design for each institution's specific simulation study using the research design, parameters, and essential elements defined by the project group; and discuss the specific and overall project goals and research with the project director during individual site visits.

Activities during the first six months of the project began with the selection of the project director and eight project sites, followed by a kickoff meeting to clarify goals and responsibilities, explore the theoretical framework for the research design, and explain the process for implementing the research over the three years of the project. After completing a comprehensive literature review to identify gaps in the simulation literature, a simulation framework was developed and the four-phase research design was formulated. Since existing measurement tools were determined to be inadequate for the purposes of this study, new research instruments were developed during Phase I.

Phase II: January 2004 to June 2004

Phase II was designed to allow each project coordinator and her faculty colleagues to have first-hand experience designing a simulation within the parameters of the framework, implementing that simulation, and evaluating its effectiveness. As a result of these efforts, study participants were able to assess what worked well, define ideal time frames for various components of the learning experience, obtain reliability and validity data on the instruments constructed to measure the concepts in the simulation teaching-learning framework, and develop a medical-surgical simulation that would be implemented across all eight sites during Phases III and IV.

Each project coordinator implemented a small simulation study at her school, with six sites using SimMan®, one site using an IV simulator, and one site using a low-fidelity mannequin. All sites used the Educational Practices in Simulation Scale (EPSS) and the Simulation Design Scale (SDS) to gather data about the experience.

The project director reviewed the curriculum at all eight sites and determined that every school taught basic care of the post-operative adult patient in the first clinical course. This content was selected, therefore, for the scenario that was designed for implementation across all sites during Phase III of the study.

Phase III: July 2004 to July 2005

Phase III consisted of two parts. Part 1 focused on obtaining baseline data about students' understanding of post-operative content before the teaching simulation was integrated. Part 2 focused on learning outcomes at the project sites when three different types of simulations were incorporated.

During Phase III, Part 1 (July to December 2004), baseline data about current practices and learning outcomes in medical-surgical courses where post-operative content is taught were obtained prior to implementing the study's simulation. The study design was then pilot tested at one site. This activity helped the group refine the simulation scenario, refine the research design, and obtain additional reliability and validity data on the instruments.

Three hundred ninety five students (female = 350; male = 45) completed a 12-item multiple choice pretest, and viewed a 38-minute videotaped lecture presented by an experienced master teacher who included a simulation of care of a post-operative adult patient. Following the lecture, students completed a 12-item parallel form post-test on post-operative care, the EPSS, the SDS, an instrument that measured their satisfaction with the instructional method, a self-confidence scale that measured their perceptions of their confidence in caring for a post-operative client, and a self-perceived judgment performance measure that provided information about students' perceptions of their clinical performance in the simulation.

In Phase III, Part 2 (January to July 2005), project sites implemented the standardized simulation focusing on care of a post-operative adult patient, using randomized control and experimental groups. Each then assessed the simulation design and process using the SDS and EPSS; each evaluated selected learning outcomes for students experiencing three different types of simulations; and each assessed student satisfaction with the use of simulation as a teaching-learning strategy. Specific research questions addressed during Phase III, Part 2 of the study were as follows:

1) Will students who participate in the simulation as part of the teaching-learning experience related to care of an adult post-operative patient have better learning outcomes (knowledge, self-confidence, satisfaction, judgment performance) based on the type of simulation experienced (paper/pencil case study simulation, static mannequin, or high-fidelity patient simulator)?

2) Will there be differences regarding learning outcomes (knowledge, self-confidence, judgment performance, and learner satisfaction) based on the role assigned to a student in the simulation?

Four hundred three students who were enrolled in their first medical-surgical nursing course participated in this phase. These students were largely female (87 percent) and Caucasian (77 percent, with 8 percent self-reporting as African American and 6 percent self-reporting as Asian), and their average age was 29. Sixty-two percent were enrolled in baccalaureate programs, and 38 percent were students in associate degree programs. All participants completed the 12-item pretest on post-operative care and viewed a 38-minute videotape that included (a) a lecture by an experienced master teacher on the care of the post-operative adult patient and (b) a simulation demonstrating care of such a patient. Students were then randomly assigned to one of three types of simulation groups, each of which focused on care of a post-operative adult patient.

- One group was given a paper/pencil case study simulation. Students worked in groups of four to answer the questions and solve the problems presented.

- A second group participated in a hands-on simulated experience using a static mannequin.

- The third group also had a hands-on experience, but they used a high-fidelity patient simulator.

All three groups were provided the same simulation, worked in groups of four, and each group's simulation was conducted for 20 minutes. All students then participated in a 20-minute reflective thinking session immediately following the simulation that was either audio taped or videotaped. This guided reflection session was facilitated by the instructor who had observed the simulation, using specific scripted questions. Students then completed the EPSS and SDS, as well as a test of their knowledge, the self-confidence scale, the judgment performance scale regarding their participation in the simulation, and a satisfaction survey.

In all instances, data collection took no longer than 30 minutes. Finally, to ensure that no students were disadvantaged because of the group to which they were assigned, all had an opportunity, prior to completion of the unit/module that included post-operative care of the adult surgical patient, to participate in the two types of simulations they had missed. None, however, took advantage of this opportunity.

Phase IV: August 2005 to June 2006

After analyzing data obtained in Phase III, the project team realized that since students only participated in one of the three types of simulations, their responses on data collection instruments were limited to the learning context they experienced (i.e., paper/pencil case study simulation, static mannequin, or high-fidelity patient simulator). Phase IV was designed, therefore, to expose all participating students to two different types of simulations, namely paper/pencil case study simulation and high-fidelity patient simulator, so they could compare the experiences. The same post-operative adult patient simulation that had been designed for Phase III of the study was used in Phase IV, and an alternate paper/pencil case study simulation was designed to parallel the high-fidelity patient simulator experience as much as possible and reflect similar content and levels of decision making. All other procedures and evaluation measures were the same as in Phase III, Part 2.

Two of the eight study sites participated in Phase IV. Half of the participating students (N = 55; 86 percent female) worked with the paper/pencil case study simulation first and then worked with the high-fidelity patient simulator. The other half of the students (N = 55; 86 percent female) participated in the simulation using the high-fidelity patient simulator first and then worked with the paper/pencil case study simulation. The following research questions guided this phase of the study:

1) Is there a difference in learner satisfaction when two different types of simulations are used by learners rather than when each student uses only one type?

2) Is there a difference in students' perceived presence and importance of educational practices when two different types of simulations are used by learners rather than when each student uses only one type?

3) Is there a difference in students' perceived presence and importance of simulation design factors when two different types of simulations are used by learners rather than when each student uses only one type?

4) Is there a difference in students' self-confidence when two different types of simulations are used by learners rather than when each student uses only one type?

5) Is there a difference in students' judgment of their performance when two different types of simulations are used by learners rather than when each student uses only one type?

The outcome measure of knowledge, using a multiple choice pre- and post-test was eliminated in this phase since nonsignificant findings were obtained in the previous study using this measure.

INSTRUMENTS

The instruments used in the project included several questionnaires, some of which were specifically designed for the study and some of which were already in existence. Each instrument is described, and content validity and reliability determined during Phase III of the study are provided for each.

The Simulation Design Scale (SDS), a 20-item instrument using a five-point scale, was designed to evaluate the five design features of the instructor-developed simulations used in this study. The five design features include objectives/information, support, problem solving, feedback, and fidelity. The instrument has two parts; one asks about the presence of specific features in the simulation, and the other asks about the importance of those features to the learner. Content validity for the SDS was established by 10 content experts in simulation development and testing. The instrument's reliability was tested using Cronbach's alpha, which was found to be 0.92 for presence of features, and 0.96 for the importance of features.

The Educational Practices in Simulation Scale (EPSS), a 16-item instrument using a five-point scale, was designed to measure whether four educational practices (active learning, collaboration, diverse ways of learning, and high expectations) are present in the instructor-developed simulation, and the importance of each practice to the learner. The educational practices were derived from the work of Chickering and Gamson (1987). Reliability was tested using Cronbach's alpha and was found to be 0.86 for the presence of specific practices and 0.91 for the importance of specific practices.

The Student Satisfaction with Learning Scale is a five-item instrument designed to measure student satisfaction with five different items related to the simulation activity. Content validity of the instrument was established by nine clinical experts validating the content and relevance of each item for the concept of satisfaction. Reliability was tested using Cronbach's alpha and found to be 0.94.

The Self-Confidence in Learning Using Simulations Scale is an eight-item instrument measuring how confident students felt about the skills they practiced and their knowledge about caring for the type of patient presented in the simulation. Content validity was established by nine clinical experts in nursing, and reliability, tested using Cronbach's alpha, was found to be 0.87.

Cognitive gain or knowledge was measured by comparing scores on multiple choice tests related to caring for a post-operative adult patient. Two parallel forms of the test were designed by a test development expert to mimic NCLEX-RN®-type questions. One form of the test was given prior to students' participation in any simulation, and the other form was given after completion of the simulation. Content validity of these tests was established by three experienced faculty.

The Self-Perceived Judgment Performance Scale is a 20-item scale modified from the Judgment Performance Scale (Facione & Facione, 1998) used to measure higher order thinking in individuals during a performance. This scale was based on students' self-perception of their performance in the simulation as scored on a five-point Likert Scale. The higher the score, the better the student perceived her/himself as performing appropriately and effectively within the simulation. Content validity of the modified scale was determined by nine clinical experts, and Cronbach's alpha established a 0.90 reliability for the scale.

Findings

Data from Phase II revealed that the prominent educational practice embedded in the simulations was that of collaboration. The most important simulation design feature was found to be feedback/debriefing.

Data from Phase III, Part I indicated that knowledge was gained by students in the traditional learning environment. Using a paired t-test, there was a significant difference ($p < .0001$) between the pre- and post-test scores, indicating learning took place. The educational practices found to be embedded in the traditional instruction were active learning, collaboration, diverse ways of learning, and high expectations. High expectations was the educational practice that received the highest rating by students indicating they perceived this educational practice to be most present in the classroom experience. Overall, students were satisfied with the traditional approach to learning about caring for a post-operative adult patient, and they indicated that this experience helped them gain confidence in their ability to care for a post-operative patient.

When comparing data obtained from the 403 students during Phase III, Part 2, responses on the Simulation Design Scale (SDS) revealed the following:

- The group that used the high-fidelity patient simulator reported a greater sense of reality than did students in the other two groups, and the paper/pencil case study simulation group reported the least sense of reality

- The group that used the paper/pencil case study simulation was less likely than the other two groups to report they received feedback, but there was no significant difference on this aspect of the simulation design in the other two groups indicating those two types of simulations (static mannequin and high-fidelity patient simulator) provide similar feedback from the instructor to students

- The groups that used the static mannequin simulation or high-fidelity patient simulator reported more opportunities to problem solve and make decisions in the simulation than did the paper/pencil case study simulation group

- Feedback was viewed as less important to the paper/pencil case study simulation group than it was to the other two groups

When comparing data obtained from the 403 students participating in Phase III, Part 2 of the study, responses on the Educational Practices in Simulation Scale (EPSS) revealed the following:

- The group that used the high-fidelity patient simulator reported a greater sense of being involved in diverse ways of learning than did students in the other two groups, and they valued this educational practice more than did students in those other groups

- The group that used the paper/pencil case study simulation agreed, more than the other two groups, that collaboration was part of their simulation

- The group that used the paper/pencil case study simulation perceived higher expectations to perform well in the learning situation than did the group that used the static mannequin simulation

- Students who participated in either simulator group (static mannequin or high-fidelity patient simulator) perceived a greater presence of active learning and rated active learning as being more important in their learning experience than did the students who worked with the paper/pencil case study simulation

When comparing data obtained from the 403 students during Phase III, Part 2, responses on the 2-item, multiple choice, NCLEX-RN®-type exam revealed that there were no significant differences in knowledge gains among the three groups as measured by pre- and post-testing, using Kruskal-Walis non-parametric tests (non-parametric version of the ANOVA) between each pair of groups. This is not a surprising finding, however, since students were not expected to acquire new knowledge during this experience. The simulations were designed to give them an opportunity to apply their knowledge, as learning with simulations should be directed toward synthesis and application of knowledge, rather than toward new knowledge development.

When comparing data obtained from the 403 students during Phase III, Part 2 of the study, responses on the Satisfaction Scale revealed that the group using the high-fidelity patient simulator had a significantly higher level of satisfaction with their learning experience than did students in the two other groups.

When comparing data obtained from the 403 students during Phase III, Part 2 of the study, responses on the Self-Confidence Scale revealed that students in the high-fidelity patient simulator and static mannequin simulation groups reported significantly greater confidence about their ability to care for a post-operative adult patient than did students in the paper/pencil case study simulation group.

When comparing data obtained from the 403 students during Phase III, Part 2 of the study, responses on the Self-Perceived Judgment Performance Scale revealed no significant difference among the three groups regarding their performance. It appears that students self-evaluate based on the context of the learning situation. If they achieved the stated objectives, and felt good about their participation, then they rated themselves as performing well.

Students who worked with the high-fidelity patient simulator or the static mannequin were randomly assigned to one of the following four roles: Nurse 1, Nurse 2, significant other, or observer. Students who participated in the paper/pencil case study simulation were not given roles. Data obtained during Phase III, Part 2 of the study revealed the following about the roles played:

- Regardless of the role they assumed during the simulation, there were no significant differences in knowledge gain among students

- Regardless of the role they assumed during the simulation, there were no significant differences in satisfaction or self-confidence regarding caring for a post-operative adult patient among students

- Students who assumed the Nurse 1 role rated themselves significantly higher on their judgment when caring for a post-operative adult patient when compared to those who assumed the Nurse 2 role

- Students who assumed the significant other role rated themselves significantly higher on their judgment when caring for a post-operative adult patient when compared to those who assumed the Nurse 2 role

- Students who assumed the observer role rated themselves significantly lower on their judgment when caring for a post-operative adult patient when compared to those who assumed the Nurse 2 role

- There were no significant differences on judgment when caring for a post-operative adult patient between those who assumed the role of Nurse 1 and those who assumed the role of significant other

When comparing data obtained from the 110 students (86 percent female; mean age of 26) who participated in Phase IV, responses on the Educational Practices in Simulation Scale (EPSS) and the Simulation Design Scale (SDS) revealed the following:

- Students in the high-fidelity patient simulator group reported active learning to be present and important significantly more often than did students in the paper/pencil case study simulation group

- Diverse ways of learning was rated higher by students in the high-fidelity patient simulator group than by those in the paper/pencil case study simulation group

- The paper/pencil case study simulation group rated collaboration and higher expectations significantly higher than did the high-fidelity patient simulator group

- The high-fidelity patient simulator group rated the importance of fidelity, presence of feedback, support, and objectives significantly higher than did the paper/pencil case study simulation group

- Overall, students in the high-fidelity patient simulator group were significantly more satisfied with their learning activity than were students in the paper/pencil case study simulation group

- The high-fidelity patient simulator group rated themselves significantly more confident and satisfied with the instruction than did the paper/pencil case study simulation group

- The paper/pencil case study simulation group judged their performance significantly higher than did the high-fidelity patient simulator group

Conclusions

Based on findings that the paper/pencil case study simulation group did not perceive as many problem solving features or opportunities to problem solve in their learning experience as the other two groups did, one can conclude that the more active the learning experience, the more important feedback is to the learner. Feedback facilitates the decision-making/problem solving process; thus, paper/pencil case study simulations may be less effective than other types of simulations in helping students develop these skills that are critical for clinical practice. Perhaps the difference can be attributed to the fact that a case study provides information about a patient while active involvement in a simulation requires students to discover and make sense of that information for themselves.

Based on findings that students in both simulator groups (i.e., static mannequin and high-fidelity) placed higher value on diverse ways of learning and active learning than did students in the paper/pencil case study simulation, one can conclude that students' judgments about the importance of various educational practices are influenced by the learning context in which they are placed. If learners are not exposed to diverse and active educational practices, they do not know what they have missed and may not value those practices.

Based on the findings that the group using the high-fidelity patient simulator had a significantly higher level of satisfaction with their learning experience than did students in the two other groups, one can conclude that high-fidelity patient simulator experiences incorporate more of the principles of best practice in education as described by Chickering and Gamson (1987).

Based on the findings that there were no significant difference among the three groups regarding their perceived performance, one can conclude that students evaluate themselves based on the context of the learning situation, not on the objectives to be attained. In other words, if they achieved the stated objectives and felt good about their participation, then they rated themselves as performing well.

Based on findings related to knowledge gain, confidence, satisfaction, and various roles assumed in a simulation (i.e., Nurse 1, Nurse 2, significant other, or observer), one can conclude that role assignment does not affect overall student learning outcomes. It is important to note that since those assigned to the observer role did not rate collaboration highly on the EPSS, faculty may need to structure the learning experience to provide some mechanism for students in this role to engage in collaborative work.

Based on findings related to student satisfaction with their learning experience, one can conclude that high-fidelity patient simulator experiences incorporate more of the principles of best practice in education as described by Chickering and Gamson (1987).

Based on findings related to self-confidence, one can conclude that learning through paper/ pencil case study simulation is not as effective in promoting confidence in students since that experience lacks realistic, timely opportunities for students to "test" themselves in providing care to patients.

Based on the findings related to performance, one can conclude that paper/pencil case study simulations may help students perceive a greater level of performance because they are more experienced with the case study method of learning.

Students who participated in paper/pencil case study simulations believed that their instructors had high expectations of them and their experience promoted collaborative learning. However, this approach provided less fidelity, fewer opportunities for problem solving, and fewer opportunities for providing feedback to students.

Overall, students who worked with the high-fidelity patient simulator were more satisfied with the instructional method and reported greater confidence in their ability to care for a post-operative adult patient. More than other students, this group believed that their experience provided for more fidelity and feedback, and they rated those design features as the most important ones. With regard to educational practices incorporated into a simulation experience, students whose experience incorporated the high-fidelity patient simulator perceived significantly more active learning and diverse ways of learning than did other students, and they rated active learning as the most important educational practice. Furthermore, these students seemed to learn and be satisfied even when they played roles other than that of "nurse" in a simulation.

Summary

The findings of this national, multi-site, multi-method study on Designing and Implementing Models for the Innovative Use of Simulation to Teach Nursing Care of Ill Adults and Children support those reported in the literature on simulations, even though that literature base is somewhat limited. It is clear that the educational practices and simulation design characteristics in the simulation framework are relevant and important to incorporate into simulations to provide a quality learning experience for students. In addition, the simulation framework has been found to be valuable as a guide for conducting systematic, organized research on simulations.

While more research is needed, it appears that immersion in a simulation provides the opportunity to apply and synthesize knowledge in a realistic but non-threatening environment. Active involvement and the opportunity to apply observational, assessment, and problem solving skills, followed by a reflective thinking experience, leads to increased self-confidence in students. In addition, when students are more active and immersed in a learning situation, the feedback they receive regarding what they did correctly and incorrectly can greatly facilitate their learning. It is expected that the expanded use of simulation in nursing education will facilitate increased learning and skill transfer when students care for patients in today's complex health care environment.

References

Chickering, A. W., & Gamson, Z. F. (1987, March). Seven principles of good practice in undergraduate education. *AAHE Bulletin, 39*(7), 5-10.

Facione, N.C., & Facione, P.A. (1998). *Professional judgment rating form*. Millbrae, CA: The California Press.